Surviving Pregnancy Loss

Surviving ❧ ❧ ❧ ❧ Pregnancy Loss

Revised and Updated

ROCHELLE FRIEDMAN, M.D.
BONNIE GRADSTEIN, M.P.H.

with a foreword by Robert H. Glass, M.D.

Little, Brown and Company
Boston   Toronto   London

Revised Edition

The authors are grateful to the *American Journal of Nursing* for
permission to quote excerpts from an article by Carol Hard-
grove and Louise Warrick entitled "How Shall We Tell the
Children," which appeared in the *American Journal of Nursing* in
March, 1974. Copyright © 1974 by the *American Journal of
Nursing*.

LIBRARY OF CONGRESS CATALOGING IN PUBLICATION DATA
Friedman, Rochelle.
    Surviving pregnancy loss.
    Bibliography: p.
    Includes index.
    1. Miscarriage—Psychological aspects. 2. Still birth—Psychological as-
pects. 3. Pregnancy, Ectopic—Psychological aspects. 4. Loss (Psychology) 5. Pregnancy—Psychological aspects. I. Gradstein, Bonnie. II.
Title.
        RG648.F74   155.9′37   82-7216
        ISBN 0-316-29396-2   AACR2

RRD VA

Published simultaneously in Canada
by Little, Brown & Company (Canada) Limited

Printed in the United States of America

Contents

Foreword

Very few pregnant women anticipate an outcome to their pregnancy that is less than perfect. Vital statistics indicate, however, that this view may be too optimistic. Fifteen of every hundred pregnancies end in a spontaneous abortion (miscarriage), another one in eighty ends in the delivery of a dead infant, while still another one in a hundred is an ectopic pregnancy. All three of these complications deprive the woman of her expected child and evoke in her and her husband feelings of loss, grief, and anger.

Unfortunately, the physician's focus on the physical problems associated with the loss of the pregnancy can interfere with his or her ability to recognize and deal with the emotional needs of the couple. A physician's usual response to a miscarriage is to inform the woman that it is a common occurrence and is nature's way of eliminating potentially abnormal individuals. This explanation, while accurate, does not deal with the couple's perception that their baby has been lost and their emotional response to that perception. Ectopic pregnancy is still a cause of maternal deaths in this country because of internal hemorrhage. For that reason, it is with a sense of relief that a physician completes the successful surgical treatment of an ectopic pregnancy. Preserving the mother's life is the paramount concern. Surgery relieves the woman of the pain associated with the ectopic pregnancy, but then she must face not only the loss of her baby, but the realization that her chances for successful pregnancy in the future are decreased substantially. Often these concerns are not addressed by physicians because of their concentration on the surgery and the physical recovery that follows it.

When confronted by pregnancy loss, friends and relatives tend to fall back on clichés that do little to assuage the couple's grief. "It's all for the best," "The baby would have been abnormal. . . ," "You'll be pregnant again soon and will have no problems" are poor substitutes for what the couple really needs — a chance to ventilate their grief. A major problem is that others do not perceive a miscarriage or ectopic pregnancy as loss of a child, whereas the couple experiences the loss often as strongly as they would the stillbirth of a full-term infant.

The response of health care professionals to the emotional needs of couples who have experienced a stillbirth has improved dramatically in the last decade. Many hospitals have specific individuals trained to help parents deal with their need to grieve and to ventilate their feelings. Follow-up sessions are provided even after the woman is discharged from the hospital, and couples are encouraged to join groups made up of individuals who have sustained similar pregnancy losses. Even with these aids couples still must rely primarily on their own psychological and emotional resources. This is especially true in today's society, where families are atomized and close relatives may be thousands of miles away.

On rare occasions a book is published that provides crucial information for both patients and their physicians. Norman Cousins's *Anatomy of an Illness* and Martha Lear's *Heartsounds* are two recent examples. *Surviving Pregnancy Loss* is another. For the individual who has suffered a pregnancy loss it shows that others have had similar experiences, similar grief, and similar emotional reactions. The book performs a vital service by bringing to the fore the realization that it is not just the wife who is traumatized. The husband too suffers and he is under the added burden of societal expectations that he will keep a stiff upper lip. This book contains not only descriptions of reactions to pregnancy loss, but also practical approaches to coping with the associated emotional problems. I cannot emphasize the last point too strongly. Couples need help, and *Surviving Pregnancy Loss* is uniquely suited to provide that help. For the physician, it will aid in understanding the emotional needs of individuals who have had a miscarriage, an ectopic pregnancy, or a stillbirth. For most physicians it will be a revelation to learn that couples can regard an ectopic pregnancy as the loss of a baby.

Let there be no mistake; the book is not a depressant. The stories told by the individuals who have lost a pregnancy are moving and evoke in the reader an admiration for the spirit of these individuals as they cope with their adversity. Moreover, the suggestions for coping provide a realistic plan for escaping the depression associated with the loss of a baby. Last, there is a wonderful chapter on adoption that demonstrates that there are alternatives even for those couples who choose not to risk the potential disappointment of another pregnancy.

In the decade since the first edition of this book was published, in vitro fertilization (IVF) and its associated technologies have become accepted medical practice. Many individuals who might not otherwise have achieved a pregnancy have overcome infertility with the aid of these techniques. But as chances for fertility have been enhanced, so too have the risks of pregnancy loss. The rate of early pregnancy loss is increased in women who conceive during IVF cycles. Spontaneous abortion rates are in the 20 to 30 percent range, and ectopic pregnancy rates are in the 3 to 5 percent range. Another problem exacerbated by the advanced reproductive technologies is that of multiple births. For most individuals, and particularly those who have had to deal with infertility, a twin pregnancy is acceptable and often welcomed. However, multiples beyond two and especially beyond three raise the specter of premature birth and its attendant adverse effects on the children. Selective abortion of excess fetuses is now a medical option, but it is a difficult choice for individuals who have had difficulty in conceiving. In addition, the procedure does entail a 10 to 25 percent chance of loss of the entire pregnancy. Although pregnancy loss with IVF represents only a small portion of the overall loss in spontaneous pregnancies, the effort, expense, and psychological commitment that accompanies IVF can make a failed pregnancy that much more difficult to bear. Moreover, the media attention focused on the successes of IVF has made the sense of failure more profound for those who either lose a pregnancy or do not achieve one.

In another area of technological and scientific advances, prenatal diagnosis and therapy directed toward the fetus in the uterus have increased the chances of successful pregnancy. At the same time, they have also magnified the need for sometimes anguished decisions over how much therapy is worthwhile and which babies can be saved to lead productive lives.

The new technologies have not eliminated pregnancy loss, and for some individuals these advances have changed their problem from infertility to spontaneous abortion, or from bearing a genetically abnormal child to deciding whether an elective abortion is preferable. This volume of *Surviving Pregnancy Loss* confronts these issues, and thus it is as timely as the first edition was in 1982. The need to realize that a miscarriage or an ectopic pregnancy can be a heartfelt loss for the parents is still acute. The need to help the parents to grieve without burdening them with clichés is still imperative.

The authors' firsthand experience with pregnancy loss is evident in these pages. Their advice is practical, concise, free of jargon, and useful for both health professionals and lay individuals. An added benefit to this volume is the updated chapter on adoption, which can be an attractive alternative to risking pregnancy loss and a means of alleviating the consequences of infertility.

Both Dr. Friedman, who is a psychiatrist, and Mrs. Gradstein, who has a master's degree in public health and is a counselor in the area of reproduction, have had extensive experience in working with couples who have experienced pregnancy loss. Their advice is sympathetic and, most important, it is practical. It also is clearly written.

Who should read this book? Everyone who has had a miscarriage, an ectopic pregnancy, or a stillbirth; anyone who has a friend or relative who has had a pregnancy loss; every physician; and, finally, anyone who wants to understand the stresses placed on the human spirit by loss of a baby, and the resiliency of individuals in coping with that misfortune.

ROBERT H. GLASS, M.D.
Professor
Obstetrics, Gynecology and Reproductive Sciences
University of California, San Francisco

Preface

Every book has a story, and every story has a beginning. *Surviving Pregnancy Loss* is somewhat unusual in that it had two beginnings. Through our own very different experiences, each of us became aware of the need for a book that would help people who had been through the loss of a pregnancy understand what had happened, cope with the loss, and plan for the future.

Dr. Rochelle Friedman's interest in working with individuals who have experienced the loss of a pregnancy dates back to the early 1970s. Until that time neither the medical nor the psychological profession had paid a great deal of attention to the many emotional and physical health problems that primarily or exclusively affect women. However, by the early 1970s that situation was starting to change in response to pressure from the women's movement as well as to increasing interest within the professions in the normal life experiences of both women and men. In this climate of opinion, old notions about women were starting to break down and a generation of articulate, concerned women was beginning to educate society about what women's health needs really were.

In 1973, one such woman, a fifty-five-year-old teacher, sought counseling for a long-standing depression. In the course of talking about her life, she recounted in minute detail the events surrounding a miscarriage she had experienced some thirty years before. Her account raised important questions: why was it that a loss so profound that it was recalled moment by moment after years had gone by been virtually ignored in medical and psychiatric training? Why had a problem that affected so many people been overlooked?

A search of the medical and lay literature confirmed the suspicion that little attention had been paid to the subject of pregnancy loss. The medical literature held only a few articles on the subject, most of them in nursing journals. The psychiatric literature was even more disappointing: all that could be found were studies and observations purporting to demonstrate that pregnancy loss is related to a woman's conflicts, whether about her femininity or about her wish for a child. As for the lay literature, there was a profusion of books that dealt with the "healthy pregnancy," but only very few that included anything at all about the complications of pregnancy or about pregnancy loss. Similarly, a fairly extensive search turned up few resources: little in the way of support services and very few health professionals who saw the need to pay attention to anything other than the physical aspects of pregnancy loss.

The decision was made to find out more about what individuals who have lost pregnancies experience and how best to meet the needs of this population. In 1976 a postmiscarriage peer support group was organized at the Massachusetts Institute of Technology, with five women participating. The group was led jointly by Dr. Friedman and Ms. Karen Cohen, then a health educator at M.I.T. The group was conceived of as being both therapeutic and educational. The goal of the educational component was to help women understand what had happened to them, so that they could achieve intellectual mastery over an event that they had initially experienced as overwhelming. The brief psychotherapy was designed to help the participants examine their experiences with pregnancy, to explore their feelings about the loss of their pregnancies, and to help them resolve their loss.

During the course of meeting together to share experiences, concerns, and support, it became clear that, although the exact circumstances of each woman's miscarriage were different from those of any other, there were many common aspects. Each of the participants had discovered that although family, friends, and medical helpers had all minimized her loss, there was a community of people who understood what they had been through. The women learned that they were not overreacting to a trivial loss, as they had been led to believe. On the contrary, they came to realize that they had been experiencing feelings of sadness and disappointment because they were mourning the loss of a specific irreplaceable and valued pregnancy.

As professionals, we learned that most women form an attachment to the fetus far earlier in the pregnancy than we had previously thought; that the child who will never be is mourned; and that the mourning process that follows the loss of a pregnancy, even an early loss, resembles that experienced when a beloved person dies. We also learned that no group of experts existed to help people through the crisis of losing a pregnancy, and, in fact, the true experts are those people who have themselves experienced such a loss. The decision to write a book by and for people who had been through this trauma developed out of this background.

Surviving Pregnancy Loss is based on clinical work with many men and women who have experienced infertility or suffered the loss of a pregnancy. It is also based on information gathered through a searching questionnaire that was completed by more than sixty women who had experienced the loss of one or more pregnancies. Participants were recruited through advertisements placed in the national newsletter of RESOLVE, an organization serving the needs of people with infertility problems, and in the national newsletter OURS, a publication of Adoptive Families of America.

In addition to the many responses, which you will find throughout this book in the form of quotations, shared experiences, and suggestions for coping, the ad yielded two completely unforeseen benefits. First, a lengthy personal narrative describing her own stillbirth was received from Charlene Arcidiacono. Reading about Mrs. Arcidiacono's experience made it clear that the best way to learn about what the loss of a pregnancy is really like is to hear about it from someone who has been through it. Mrs. Arcidiacono's account can be found in the section on stillbirth, "One Woman's Experience."

The "request for contact" notice in the RESOLVE newsletter also yielded a telephone call from Bonnie Gradstein, a woman who was deeply interested and involved in the area of pregnancy loss. In addition to having lost two pregnancies herself, she was a professional counselor who often dealt with other women who were coping with pregnancy loss. After many hours on the phone between Boston and San Francisco, it became clear to both of us that we had to write this book together. Thus our collaboration began.

Mrs. Gradstein's belief that a book about what it was really like to lose a pregnancy was long overdue, her vast experience in the field of reproductive-health counseling, and her own experiences make her the natural person to collaborate on the kind of book that she wishes had been available to her when she needed it.

Mrs. Gradstein acquired a firsthand knowledge of how lonely, baffling, and agonizing the loss of a pregnancy could be when her first pregnancy ended in miscarriage and her second with the birth of a stillborn child. Although she was lucky in many respects, for her family and friends were loving and supportive, for the first time in her life she felt totally alone, empty, and out of control. She remembers walking around in a fog, sad and uncomprehending, wondering why she felt so bad, if she was crazy, and if her life was really falling apart. Although she managed to survive the experience, it was the hardest thing she had ever had to face. The struggle was a lonely one: there was nothing out there to help her — no books to read, no one to tell her she would make it.

As a result of these two losses, the focus of her career as a counselor changed significantly. Whereas in the past most of the women she had worked with had gone on to have healthy babies, now she was led to try to meet the needs of a different group, one for whom there was no existing support system: couples who had problems with having babies, some who had difficulty conceiving and others who were unable to carry a pregnancy to term.

Also, as a result of their own experience in adopting a child, Mrs. Gradstein and her husband, Marc, a practicing attorney, learned a great deal about private adoption. With the encouragement and support of the Department of Obstetrics, Gynecology and Reproductive Sciences at the University of California, San Francisco, for the past fifteen years they have been educating people about private adoption, as well as guiding many through the private adoption process.

ROCHELLE FRIEDMAN
BONNIE GRADSTEIN

Introduction

Despite medical advances, every pregnancy does not produce a healthy child. Things can and do go wrong. Unfortunately, about one in five pregnancies is lost: approximately one in five women suffers a miscarriage, one in eighty pregnancies ends in the birth of a stillborn child, and 1 to 2 percent of all pregnancies are ectopic. Still other pregnancies are terminated when prenatal diagnosis reveals that the fetus has serious difficulties. About one million women a year in this country have an unsuccessful pregnancy.

The loss of a baby is almost always unforeseen. Although pregnancy loss is not uncommon, it is understandable that pregnant women most often choose not to focus on the possibility. It is a frightening possibility, one that is safer to keep below the surface, in the back of one's mind. "Why should I worry about something that probably will not happen?" is a common reaction. Therefore, when it does happen, it usually comes as a shock, and the woman is unprepared for both the physical and the emotional aftermath. Following pregnancy loss, women are often faced with unexplained feelings and find that they have trouble coping with what has happened. They commonly feel that they have nowhere to turn for help.

Surviving Pregnancy Loss is designed to address the needs of women who have experienced miscarriage, stillbirth, ectopic pregnancy, or selective termination secondary to a poor outcome on prenatal diagnostic procedures. Its goal is to help women understand the medical and psychological aspects of what has happened to them and how they are feeling about it. To this end, we have included not only a description of what one typically experiences when a pregnancy is lost, but also, wherever possible, up-to-date medical information about each specific type of loss. In addition, we have drawn widely both upon available knowledge about human behavior and on our own clinical experience in order to give a framework for ordering and understanding these experiences. Lastly, we have included concrete suggestions for coping as well as help in planning for the future.

While this book is not written specifically for women who have had voluntary abortions, we recognize that they may experience feelings similar to those of women who have lost desired pregnancies. Particularly relevant are the sections of this book that address the complex feelings of attachment and yearning that often develop even early in pregnancy and the sections that examine the feelings of grief experienced when pregnancy is lost.

Our clinical experience has shaped the content and organization of this book. We begin with an overview in which we take a look at the feelings a woman is likely to have during and after the loss of a baby. We then describe each type of loss: miscarriage, stillbirth, ectopic pregnancy, and selective termination. Even though most readers will have already experienced a pregnancy loss, we have found that it is a critical part of the mourning process to relive the experience; thus the book includes, for each type of loss, a description of the physical experience, a discussion about causes, treatment, and recovery, and a personal account: one woman's story. In addition, each chapter describes emotional reactions unique and specific to that loss. The discussion of each loss is likely to stir memories, trigger conversations, and help the woman understand why the impact of her loss was so great. For those women who have experienced the loss of more than one pregnancy, we have also included a chapter on multiple losses.

We go on to describe the effect of the loss on the woman's partner and to present a personal account of one man's experience. The husband's experience is different in many ways from that of his wife. His emotions and behavior are often misunderstood: this can become a source of conflict in the marriage. The effect on the marital relationship of losing a pregnancy is covered in detail, including cautions, pitfalls to avoid, and suggestions for coping. We then focus on the impact of the loss on other children and on family and friends.

We conclude with "Planning for the Future," a section that we hope enables the reader to look toward the future — a future that may include the options of becoming pregnant again, choosing to remain childless, or deciding to adopt. This chapter is designed to give the reader specific information about each option as well as to help her decide which alternatives best suit her and her partner.

We have included a lengthy chapter on adoption because we view it as a particularly attractive option for those who are not biologically able to have a child, as well as for those who do not want to risk another disappointment or live with continual uncertainty. Our experience leads us to conclude that if a couple choose to become parents, the future can hold children for them, whether by birth or adoption.

We suggest that you use the book in the following way. We recommend that everyone read the first section, which deals with the emotional impact of losing a baby. If you have experienced one of the four types of loss, we suggest you read the chapter that applies to you. If you have experienced more than one type, you may want to read more than one chapter as well as chapter 7 on multiple losses.

We encourage you to read any other chapter that interests you. We do not anticipate that every reader will read every chapter. The goal of this book is not just to educate you, but to help you think about your experience and begin putting it into perspective. We suggest you think about the book as a time line. It can facilitate thinking about the past, coping with the present, and looking toward the future. You may choose to read some chapters now and save others for some future time.

Some readers may wonder why we have included chapters on trying again, adoption, and childlessness. The healing process necessarily takes women into the future and these chapters will provide some of the information they are looking for.

We hope this book will be particularly interesting and useful, too, to families and friends close to those who have lost a pregnancy, as well as to professionals such as doctors, midwives, nurses, social workers, members of the clergy, and others who have contact with people affected by this loss. We anticipate that reading this book will heighten their awareness of the impact that losing a pregnancy can have, and that it will enable them to provide needed support and understanding. In addition, we hope that they will recommend this book to those affected, as a means of helping them in their struggle.

I

The Experience of Losing a Pregnancy 🐾 🐾 🐾 🐾

"If I could want people who haven't lost a pregnancy to know one thing, it would be to know that it is a real loss. It's not just easy like stubbing your toe. It can be physically painful, like labor. It's not just like having your period. It's the death of a child. It doesn't matter that you can have another, although that is not always true. This particular child is gone and will never come again. You will love the baby you adopt or give birth to in the future, but that is not the child whose loss you have a right to mourn."

1

The Emotional Impact

THE NATURE OF THE ATTACHMENT

All of us come to the decision to have children in our own ways. Some of us have looked forward to parenthood since we were children, while others have come to this choice only later in our lives. Some of us have chosen to have children early in our marriages or before starting a career; others have elected to postpone having children until marriage or career were well under way. Whatever the particular path you traveled to come to this decision, it is likely that once it was made, you became emotionally invested in carrying out your goal.

Pregnancy is a time of hopes, fantasy, and preparation for the future. As you eagerly anticipate the arrival of a child, you psychologically prepare yourself for what life will be like. You imagine what it will be like to hold, feed, or bathe a baby; to see his first smile or witness her first step, and you imagine what it will be like to be a parent.

Concrete preparations are also necessary. If childless, you must prepare yourself for a major change in your life-style. If you already have children, you must tell them about the expected arrival of a new brother or sister; in addition, you need to make plans for coping with the added responsibility that another child will bring. Expectant parents may ready themselves for the new baby by moving to a larger home, stopping or cutting back on work, or arranging for child care. Names may be chosen, a nursery readied, and baby clothes and equipment purchased.

Most people experience pregnancy as a major life event. Some see becoming pregnant as "coming of age," as a confirmation of their passage from childhood to adulthood; while others see it as the fulfillment of themselves as men or women. Whatever the symbolic meaning that it may have had for you, it is likely that losing your pregnancy has influenced where you experience yourself to be in the life cycle. Some couples find themselves extremely frustrated by the discrepancy between their wish to be parents, their readiness to be parents and Nature's failure to comply. They feel eager to move on to the next step in their lives and to take on the responsibility of caring for a dependent being, but they are thwarted in their desire.

For many couples, having a baby is part of a larger life plan. Whether their goal was to bring a child into their lives, create a family, carry on a bloodline, or strengthen a relationship, the loss of a pregnancy deprives them of the possibility of achieving their goal this time. This leaves many couples feeling they are in limbo. They have left one life stage behind, and the next seems to be eluding them. It is most likely that the woman will be able to conceive another pregnancy, carry it without difficulty, and deliver a healthy baby. However, as evidenced by their present situation, there are no guarantees. Those who have had difficulty conceiving, who have lost other pregnancies, or who have had their fertility impaired following an ectopic pregnancy may be particularly concerned about ever being able to have the child they want.

Deciding to have a child is the first step in the process of attachment. Initially we are pulled by a fantasy of ourselves as parents, a vision, if the pregnancy is our first, of what life will be like with a child. We might visualize how our lives will change with another child if we already have one or more. When we do become pregnant our dream promises to come true, and we allow ourselves to become even more attached to a vision of a different future and to the child we are carrying.

Pregnancy is a unique state; it is the only time in life when you are carrying another life within you. On a quite literal level you are not living for yourself alone. On a psychological level it is common to experience the child within you both as part of yourself and as a separate being. It is normal and healthy to feel emotionally fused with the baby you are carrying. During pregnancy you become the center of your own private world, guarding the precious life within. Outside matters touch you differently than they did previously. Feeling that the pregnancy is central to your life and that most of your emotional resources are focused on it is also quite normal. In fact, your ability to visualize yourself as a mother and to form an attachment to the child you are carrying is critical to forming a healthy relationship with your child.

In our clinical experience we have found that it is not unusual for women who wanted to be pregnant and who desired to have a child to experience second thoughts or misgivings, once they are pregnant, about what they have gotten themselves into. This observation has been borne out by two studies that examined how women adjust to pregnancy. Both found that it is quite normal to experience some ambivalent feelings about being pregnant. In addition to being an exciting and gratifying experience, pregnancy, particularly a problem pregnancy, can be uncomfortable, stressful, and even, at times, somewhat frightening.

The woman who finds that she does not like some or all aspects of being pregnant may feel guilty. If the pregnancy is successful her negative feelings are eventually minimized, forgotten, or overshadowed by the positive outcome. Such, however, is often not the case if the pregnancy fails. Then the woman may feel that her ambivalent feelings about being pregnant, about having a child, or about being a mother contributed in some way to the unfortunate outcome of her pregnancy.

Sometimes, however, the loss of a pregnancy highlights the other pole of the mother's ambivalence. It is not unusual to find women who, although initially uncertain about whether they wanted to have a child, no longer are so. These individuals find that the experience of being pregnant and losing the pregnancy has helped them discover how much they really want what they have lost.

The bond that a mother forms to her unborn child is unique. Usually you form an attachment to others on the basis of your love of the other's distinct self and because of his or her relationship to you. In pregnancy, you may feel an attachment to a fetus who is not known to you in the usual way that others in your life are known. The pregnant mother brings a lifetime of experience of knowing, loving, and caring for others to this new and unique relationship.

At first her attachment is to a fantasy image of her future child. She loves a hoped for, longed for child. She may imagine what the baby will look like, what sex it will be, and perhaps even give it a name.

As pregnancy progresses, the mother forms an actual acquaintance with her child, not through the usual ways we come to know others in our lives, but through physical sensations: the baby's weight inside her, its contours and movements. As the fetus grows and becomes more active, the mother increasingly experiences it as separate from herself.

At delivery, the mother is physically separated from her child. It is also necessary for her to cope with psychological separateness: her baby is now a unique being and must be loved as separate from herself. When the birth process proceeds normally, the mother loses the child inside her while gaining an "outside" real baby. When pregnancy fails or a stillbirth occurs, there is both the loss of the child the mother had grown to know and love and the loss of the one she imagined it would someday become. In addition, there will be no baby to compensate for the loss of the internally experienced child.

Attachment begins at different times in the pregnancy for different women. Even for the same women the attachment process is often somewhat different from one pregnancy to another. Commonly women who have already had a successful pregnancy form an attachment to their future child earlier in the next pregnancy than does an inexperienced mother: they trust that being pregnant will lead to having a child. In contrast, women who have had the experience of losing a pregnancy often find themselves holding back on forming an emotional attachment: they may treat pregnancy as a "condition" and may not allow themselves to think about the child inside them, so as to protect themselves from the pain of loss should the pregnancy fail. Similarly, women who are planning on having prenatal diagnostic procedures such as amniocentesis or ultrasound often inhibit themselves from forming an attachment until they are certain that the fetus is normal.

THE NATURE OF LOSS

Why is the loss of a pregnancy so painful? How can you mourn someone you never knew, something that the world tells you was not a baby? Your doctor may have said something like: "It's all for the best — this is nature's way of assuring that only healthy babies are born." He or she has told you that you can try again in a few months. Then, why does it seem as if your entire life has come to a screeching halt? Why the excruciating grief and yearning that you feel?

The grief that you felt and perhaps still feel when your pregnancy was lost is not as puzzling a response as is often thought. Soon after conception the psychological and physiological processes of pregnancy are set into motion. The level of reproductive hormones in your circulation increases greatly, your uterus develops a thick lining to support the growing fetus, and your breasts enlarge in preparation for nursing. The aim of these processes is to prepare both your body and your psyche for your expected child. When a pregnancy is lost this preparation is interrupted, and you are left in a state of physical and emotional readiness for a baby that will never be.

It is possible, and in fact quite common, to experience a great deal of pain after losing a pregnancy that in actuality had no possibility of succeeding, as with an ectopic pregnancy, or with a "blighted ovum," where the severe nature of the genetic defect makes life impossible. How can one form an attachment to something that was really only a small mass of undifferentiated tissue? The answer to this question is central to understanding why you are feeling so much pain, as well to explaining why the loss feels different to you than to anyone else. Early in pregnancy you formed a mental image of the child you were carrying; this image was a composite of your hopes and wishes and maybe also of your fears. Usually this process begins well before anything remotely like a baby is present. Because your feelings for your future child began before there was a child, and because they grew independently of any actual fetal development, they have a life of their own. This does not make them any less significant — after all, in other areas of life one has hopes and expectations; and one is sorely disappointed when one's dreams are shattered.

Many factors influence how you experience the loss of a pregnancy. Among these are whether or not the pregnancy was consciously desired, whether or not you already have another child, your age, the length of time you have been trying to have a baby, and whether or not you have lost earlier pregnancies.

Also significant is whether you had formed an attachment to your future child at the time when your pregnancy was lost. Once the bonding process has begun, the loss of your pregnancy is likely to be quite painful. Pain is experienced on many levels. Foremost there is the loss of your beloved child; there are also the frustration of your hopes for yourself, the loss of your pregnancy, and the denial of your wish to be a parent.

If your loss occurred late in pregnancy, after you had felt your baby kick and move, or seen it on ultrasound, or heard its heart sounds during visits to your doctor, the sense of loss that you feel is likely to be intense. You have lost a real baby in addition to a dream. With a late loss you grieve for a baby that you have lived with and loved for many months.

In the months following the loss of a pregnancy, people often ask themselves why they are so upset. This is because many of us may be totally unfamiliar with either the kinds of feelings that we are having, or with feelings of such intensity. Moreover, we may be puzzled by our reaction because we don't understand the true nature of the loss we have experienced.

Because you and your future child shared the most intimate of relationships for a period of time, it is likely that the loss of your pregnancy evoked many of the same feelings you have had when a person whom you have loved has died. This is because for you the fetus was a child and the loss of your pregnancy or of your stillborn baby was a death.

The individual who has lost a beloved person usually experiences several stages of grief. Women who have experienced pregnancy loss commonly go through a parallel grief process. Although the internal experience of loss is essentially the same in both situations, mourning following the loss of a pregnancy differs in several ways from that which occurs after a death. When a fetus is lost there is no tangible "outside" person to mourn, and mourning someone who is not physically present is known to be particularly difficult. In addition, because there are no memories and no shared life experiences the loss often has a feeling of unreality about it.

Contributing to this feeling of unreality is the commonly described experience of finding that the attachment one feels toward one's future child may not be shared by anyone else, even one's spouse. There are many reasons why this is so. Especially when the loss has occurred early in the pregnancy, the mother may be the only one who knows that she is pregnant. She alone at this point has an awareness that something special is happening inside her. This awareness makes the pregnancy "real" for her; thus when the pregnancy is lost she knows that she has lost something, while others have a hard time recognizing that anything much has happened.

While a prospective father may share his wife's desire for a child, the fact that the pregnancy is not part of his physical self makes the experience less immediate, and often less real, for him. One consequence is that the father may feel little or no attachment to his future child until late in the pregnancy, or even not until it is born. Consequently, when the pregnancy is lost in the early months, or even later, as with a stillbirth, the father may not yet have formed an attachment to his child, and so may not mourn its passing as intensely.

Friends, relatives, and even your physician may not understand what the loss of your pregnancy means to you. They did not share your experience and so are probably unaware of the depth of your feelings for your yet unborn child. Because they did not experience the attachment that you felt that may not be able to appreciate your pain, or even understand it, so they may be able to offer you little in the way of support. You may be made to feel that your emotional reactions are inappropriate or excessive, or you may be encouraged to bottle up your feelings and behave as if nothing has happened.

Before you are persuaded to write yourself off as hysterical, unstable, or a failure at coping, keep in mind that in our culture most people are uncomfortable with grief: they have difficulty dealing with strong feelings in others and/or tolerating those same feelings in themselves. It is important to remember that it is *their* inability to tolerate strong, painful feelings that is the problem, and that your feelings are a normal reaction to the loss you have suffered.

When we lose a beloved person, society recognizes the appropriateness of grieving and offers us various social rituals which help us cope with the death. We are permitted to grieve and mourn, and often others mourn with us. When a woman loses a pregnancy, she is confronted by a unique dilemma: although she may feel that she has lost something precious, she may receive little support for these feelings. Many women have felt that one of the most painful aspects of losing a pregnancy was that others in their life were unable to appreciate the extent to which they felt bereaved by their loss.

The loss of a pregnancy is a life crisis that is largely ignored by modern society: the fetus is regarded as a nonperson, and its loss as a nonevent. Society denies the importance of what has happened and discourages the expression of grief by letting the woman know that she didn't really lose anything; she can always try again soon.

GRIEF AND MOURNING

Some women experience severe grief at the loss of a pregnancy; others feel disappointment that is less marked. It is not unusual to mourn for weeks or months after losing a pregnancy or having a stillborn child. It is important to remember that mourning is a slow, painful, but important process of coping with loss. It is not only acceptable to grieve; grieving must take place before healing can occur.

Although not everyone reacts to loss in the way you do, there are some aspects of mourning that are commonly experienced. The initial stage of the grief process is frequently one of emotional numbness and disbelief. Gradually, the full impact of what has happened sinks in, and numbness gives way to a period of active mourning, which may last anywhere from several weeks to many months. During this period one is apt to feel sad, emotionally unstable, and somewhat irritable; may cry easily and at the slightest provocation; may be preoccupied with the loss and uninterested in the outside world, and may prefer to avoid contact with anyone or anything that reminds one of the loss. Contrary to popular expectations, a woman probably won't bounce right back and be herself again:

healing takes much longer than one might anticipate. Finally the pain lessens and one is able to go on with life.

Each person must progress through the mourning process in his or her own way. How you experience and express grief in response to pregnancy loss is determined by many factors, including how you usually handle feelings, how you characteristically deal with stress, whether or not you have experienced other losses, how supportive your spouse is, how your social network reacts, what else is going on in your life at the time, and what your prognosis for future success in childbearing is.

Also important are the actual circumstances of your loss. Shock may be particularly severe if you were suddenly confronted by the knowledge that your pregnancy was doomed or that your child had died. Likewise, if you were physically exhausted from labor, the initial impact of the loss may have been overwhelming. Possibly there were indications all along that the pregnancy was in trouble. If this was the case for you, it is likely that you had prepared yourself for the possibility that there might be difficulty and had begun to grieve in advance.

It is not unusual for mourners to deny the death for a brief period of time. It seems too much for them to comprehend and they feel emotionally frozen, apathetic, or confused: reactions that indicate that they cannot deal with the loss at present. When fetal death is diagnosed before labor begins, the couple may still hope that the doctor is wrong, that somehow the baby is alive. Even after the delivery, some parents may find it difficult to believe that their child has died.

Nancy, in her late twenties, said: "I had been so happy with my pregnancy — I enjoyed growing big and feeling the baby move. After the delivery of our stillborn daughter, I felt strange. The baby I carried for eight months, who was so much a part of me, my life, my thoughts, was gone. I felt so empty. The first day I kept touching my stomach, I guess to help me feel through my sense of touch, that it was real — my baby was gone. I cried that day but mostly felt numb."

As the reality of the death sinks in, it is common to experience feelings of disappointment, sadness, and yearning. The emotional pain that you feel may be so intense that it feels like a physical sensation: tightness in your chest, a knot in the pit of your stomach, or a feeling of being empty inside. Initially you may not be able to stop crying. Tears may flow continuously, or the pain may come in waves. The sadness that you feel seems to emerge from deep within you, and the tears that flow down your face and the sobs that escape from your throat seem to have bubbled up from a place within you that you didn't know existed. It is not unusual to feel preoccupied with thoughts of one's lost child, and isolated from the rest of the world by grief. For a while, one feels like an observer, a wooden doll who goes through the motions of living but feels nothing.

You may develop specific fears or feel generally anxious. Life feels very fragile after a loss, and it is sometimes difficult to prevent one's concern from spreading. You may fear for your own well-being, your husband's, your parents', or that of other children. For a while it may feel as if danger is everywhere, and as if no one you love is ever safe.

Intense sadness or depression may be accompanied by physical symptoms such as fatigue, listlessness, inability to concentrate, loss of appetite, and difficulty in sleeping. You may feel as if you have no energy, as if the smallest effort is too much for you. Since you don't feel like doing anything for a while, you sit in a chair or lie in bed for hours at a time. Sometimes entire days may slip by that way. You may find that you eat only because others tell you to. Food has no taste, and swallowing is hard because you have a lump in your throat.

You may find yourself unable to take pleasure in people, things, or activities that you previously enjoyed, and you may find that you prefer being alone to being with other people. Nothing seems to help, no one understands, and everyone says either too little or the wrong thing. Worst of all, your mind keeps returning to your loss: you review everything that happened and reexperience all of the pain all over again. You find yourself trying to figure out why it happened, and you try first one explanation, then another, then another.

At first everything is a reminder, a song on the radio, babies on television commercials, babies smiling up at you from the pages of every magazine and newspaper. It seems as if pregnant women are everywhere, as if everyone you know is either pregnant or just had a baby.

Often bedtime is the worst time of all. You may experience difficulty falling asleep and difficulty staying asleep. It seems to take you hours to fall asleep; then when you finally manage to doze off you are able to sleep only briefly and fitfully. Frequently women remark that their sleep is disturbed by nightmares. Sometimes the nightmare returns night after night, as was Margery's experience: "I had a terrible recurring nightmare for a year in which the fetus wasn't really dead but was stuck in a bottle of formaldehyde in a closet in the hospital. It was crying, 'Mommy, Mommy, I'm here. Come and get me.' I kept running down the halls, opening closets, and could never find it, even though I saw it in my mind."

For a while your emotions may be so intense, so painful, and so frightening that you may think you will never feel anything else; you may even fear that you are losing your mind. Rest assured; as time passes the pain will gradually fade and you will begin to feel better. However, don't anticipate that the climb back will be a steady one. More often, the months after losing a pregnancy are something like a ride on a roller coaster. You may find that after an initial period during which you experience an unremitting depression, your moods seem to fluctuate widely; one moment you are feeling pretty good; the next, you are in the depths of despair. While normally it takes quite a lot to throw you off balance, in the months following your loss almost anything can destroy your fragile sense of control. Any small thing can trigger the pain all over again. Sometimes you will be aware of what precipitated it; on other occasions you might find that you have plummeted back into a depression for no obvious reason.

In addition to feelings of grief, bereaved people may find themselves having a variety of other painful and perplexing emotions. You may find that you feel unusually irritable and upset by things. Some women report an unusually low tolerance level, while others feel themselves oversensitive to real or imaginary slights. You may discover that you react irritably or with anger to incidents that would not ordinarily bother you and, although you are aware that your reactions are irrational, you are unable to stop yourself. Chances are that you are feeling as if something outside you has taken over your formerly reasonable self. In fact, one probably significant impact on the way you are feeling is that you are experiencing hormone withdrawal. The level of progesterone in a woman's circulation drops markedly anywhere from several weeks to a few days before a pregnancy is actually lost. Although there is not complete agreement, many physicians feel that the rapid decrease in reproductive hormone levels that occurs as the time of delivery approaches may be responsible for causing alterations in mood, including a predisposition to depression, anxiety, and irritability.

Unfortunately, this physiological stress hits you at a time when you are both physically and emotionally vulnerable, and so already compromised in your ability to cope. One result of this stress overload is to overtax your normal coping mechanism, leaving you feeling helpless, out of control, and overwhelmed. When this happens, you may well rely on more primitive or infantile ways of dealing with the world than is usual for you, anger being one such way. It seems as if there is an unhappy coincidence of events — the actual loss of the pregnancy, reproductive hormone withdrawal, and stress overload — all of which are apt to leave you with an unusually low threshold for feeling angry.

One woman commented, "I felt numb, depressed, angry, upset and shaky, and disoriented until I got home. At home, I felt numb, tired, and angry for a few months. I felt many times 'How could this happen to me?' "

The most likely recipients of your anger are those whom you are close to — your spouse, friends, relatives, your obstetrician, or even God. You may be feeling angry with them for things that they did or didn't do, or your anger with them may be more generalized. Your tendency to be easily irritated may lead you to magnify insults, or to misinterpret well-intentioned behavior.

The anger that you feel toward others may also stem from sources other than your irritable state. Sometimes the anger that you feel toward other people in your life results from a projection or a displacement of your own feelings onto them, as when you end up blaming your obstetrician for something that was out of his control. This is not to imply that all the anger you feel is irrational. It is quite probable that you will run into people who minimize your loss and others who treat you in a thoughtless or insensitive manner.

Feelings of guilt often torment both parents. Most people find it difficult to cope with events that are beyond their control and that they do not understand. We are used to living in a world where things happen for a specific reason. However, if you are among the vast majority of couples who have lost a pregnancy, it is likely that the cause of your loss either was not sought, or, if sought, could not be determined. You probably have been unable to learn very much about what happened to you, and you may have had to rely on your fantasies about what might have gone wrong.

In their search for a plausible explanation, many couples find that they keep reviewing the period of the pregnancy before the onset of difficulty for evidence of something that may have gone wrong or that they may have done wrong. A related preoccupation may be reviewing the pregnancy to see possible missed opportunities for preventing the loss. As one woman said, "It is hard to feel that there isn't a reason. I know that the fetus was possibly abnormal, but I still keep on thinking about whether I did anything to cause my miscarriage."

In some cases couples carry a burden of guilt related to a past event: a previous therapeutic abortion, premarital sex, promiscuity, an extramarital affair, or even to sexual practices or fantasies. Sometimes one or both partners may feel guilty for feeling ambivalent about the pregnancy. They may blame themselves for causing their own difficulties and feel that the failure of the pregnancy was a punishment to teach them a lesson.

Annette, a teacher, commented, "I tried to figure out what I did to cause it. Was I too tense during the pregnancy; was that it? Did I eat right? Did I do too much? Was I too sexually active? The doctor would give me no answers."

Many couples find that their own tendency to search for causes and to blame themselves is reinforced by much of society's mythology about pregnancy loss. Everyone has a theory about what may have caused your difficulties. Usually, the theory is shared in the hopes that you will be able to make use of the information and do things differently next time. Nevertheless, it is sometimes difficult to avoid feeling that you are being blamed and to keep from holding yourself responsible.

Patricia found her own way to cope. "When someone makes a comment, I usually say something like, 'If the fetus could not take the stress of everyday living, it was not meant to survive.' I read that in a book and memorized it. I have no intentions of spending the entire nine months of my next pregnancy (see how optimistic I am?) flat on my back, which some have suggested. If someone persists, I intend to say calmly, 'Are you trying to make me feel guilty?' "

The endless cycle of uncertainty, blame, and guilt can be exhausting. Couples who get trapped in this cycle do so because they devote themselves to resolving the uncertainty by searching for an explanation of what happened. Because this is unlikely to be fruitful, their anxiety grows and their need to know what happened may increase even more.

Fortunately, there are several ways out of this predicament. The simplest solution is to come to terms with the unhappy reality that there are things in life that *are* beyond your control. Easily said, but hard to accept. While you are struggling with this issue, it may be useful to think about what you can do to decrease the anxiety that you feel. Several things that others have found helpful are finding a supportive, caring physician, speaking to other women who have lost pregnancies, and sharing their feelings with their husbands. Discussions with such people about real and mythical causes of pregnancy loss should be helpful in alleviating your own concerns.

A reaction that may surprise and dismay you is your envy of women who have children or who are pregnant. It is not unusual for women who have lost a pregnancy to feel singled out by fate and envious of others who appear to be more fortunate. Many women with whom we have spoken have found that they were unable to see a pregnant woman without feeling acutely jealous. More than one woman told of being warned by her husband when a pregnant woman was approaching on the street, so that she could avert her gaze, and so avoid bursting into tears. As one woman said: "It's not exactly that I want what they have; it's just that I want to have a baby too, and sometimes the wanting is so painful that I can't stand it."

Many woman find it extremely upsetting to learn that friends or relatives have become pregnant or that they have delivered healthy babies. One woman said: "I wanted to be big and swollen and instead I was empty. My sister-in-law was pregnant and I didn't want to see her. My husband's family said practically nothing about our stillbirth, but my mother-in-law would give me progress reports on my sister-in-law's pregnancy. Her insensitivity hurt me deeply. And I was envious and bitter at my sister-in-law's healthy pregnancy."

Judy, a pretty, dark-haired woman who miscarried in the third month of pregnancy for the second time, found herself hating all of her pregnant friends. "I felt so awful about the way that I felt; I was so filled with sadness, jealousy, and anger. I even wished that my best friend, who had become pregnant at about the same time that I did, would miscarry, too. I just couldn't stand to see her afterwards, even though she was empathetic and tried her best to be helpful to me. I just hated her because she had what I wanted and that was that. I know it was irrational, but that's how I felt."

If being with pregnant women or with couples who have small children is very painful, you may want to avoid these encounters for a while. Most people will understand if you explain to them why you are not able to speak to them by phone or be with them for now. A simple explanation should suffice such as: since you lost your pregnancy it has been difficult for you to have contact with anyone or anything that reminds you of your loss.

In the aftermath of losing a pregnancy, some women experience feelings of inadequacy. Many women with whom we have spoken have expressed concerns about their femininity, their bodily functioning, and their capacity to have children. They see other women as competent and complete while they see themselves as inadequate and damaged. They see their failure to produce a healthy baby as evidence of their failure as women.

A woman who had such feelings said, "I had a very difficult time letting friends know that I had a miscarriage. I was embarrassed. I seemed to think I had failed and that other people's knowing about it would make me ashamed. I also hated myself and my body. I thought my body had betrayed me and I could not trust it anymore. This terrible feeling still bothers me."

An often-encountered manifestation of these concerns is the anxiety that many women experience about their ability to become pregnant again. This anxiety is understandable in the case of women who have previously had difficulty conceiving. However, it is not unusual for women who have not had this problem to worry about whether they will be able to get pregnant again.

"Mentally, I was becoming obsessed with conception," Joyce said. "I was not really interested in much else. I gradually began to believe we would never have children, but I couldn't quit trying month after month."

Not uncommonly, this concern becomes increasingly intense as attempts to conceive again are not met with success. Eileen started to try to conceive again after her third normal menstrual period. Even though she had conceived her first pregnancy in the first month of trying, she was doubtful of her ability to become pregnant again. As several months passed and she still was not pregnant, her concern reached panic proportions and she sought counseling help. Eileen described how in the months since her miscarriage becoming pregnant again had become the focus of her life. "I lived by my basal temperature chart. We had intercourse at the prescribed times even when we didn't feel like it and even if it meant that my husband had to make up an excuse to get out of going out of town. As the end of my cycle neared, my anxiety mounted. It got so that I could not think of anything else. I would go into the bathroom every hour or so to see if I had started bleeding. I interpreted every twitch of pain in my pelvis as either a good omen or a bad one, depending on my mood. I stared endlessly at my chart in an attempt to divine which way the line would be going next. Needless to say, I was not much fun to live with during all of this. Sometimes I wonder how my husband put up with me. The worst time was usually the first day of my period. Then everything looked hopeless. I was sure that there was something wrong with me and I was convinced that I would never have a child."

Most women regard the renewal of their menstrual cycle in the months following their loss as evidence that their bodies have returned to normal. But, like Eileen, those anxious to conceive again often find themselves sad and disappointed with a renewed sense of personal failure with each subsequent period. For many, menstruation is seen as painful evidence of their nonpregnant state, a symbol of their inadequacy and either consciously or unconsciously associated with the lost pregnancy.

A sense of inadequacy may spread beyond the realm of biological functioning for some women. They experience the loss as evidence of their more generalized inferiority and worthlessness. Feelings of inadequacy, loss of attractiveness, physical inferiority, and lack of productiveness can overshadow their previously sound sense of self-worth. A woman who went through this said, "I felt my body was inadequate, inferior, that there was something wrong with it. My husband's disappointment over our loss made me feel I had let him down. The stillbirth colored my whole view of myself. I was negative about myself — I felt worthless, incompetent. From being an out-going, happy young woman, I became sullen and withdrawn. It took time to build up my confidence again, but I gradually did, with help from my husband."

COPING

In the months following the loss of your pregnancy, some uncomfortable confrontations may be in store for you. Other women who have survived this difficult time have offered suggestions about how to manage.

First, because a nursery full of baby clothes and furnishings may trigger painful feelings, many couples prefer to pack these things away. Others may leave everything as it is in the hope that they will eventually have a baby. You may decide that you would prefer someone else to pack away the baby things before you arrive home from the hospital. On the other hand, doing this yourself may be a way to mourn your loss, or a way to grasp the reality and finality of it. You may want your husband, a family member, or a friend to tell others the bad news for you, or you may want to let people know by yourself. In either case, be prepared to face questions from people who haven't heard. Acquaintances who are unaware of your experience may ask such questions as "How old is your baby now?" "Was it a girl or a boy?" or they may offer congratulations. You may wish to rehearse how you will handle telling your bad news. Although you will probably feel sad each time this happens, you may also find that others can offer you comfort, understanding, and support.

"It was helpful to have people to talk to. I hated being alone. Everyone's obvious sympathy really helped me a lot. No one made light of my grief — no platitudes about how I'd have a baby soon.

Instead, more of 'This must be very hard for you.' At home, my friends who'd had miscarriages were great. They really understood the most. One friend who visited started to cry. I cried. We talked and cried for about two hours. When she left, I felt great."

There are certain times, places, events, and people that are certain to be difficult to confront for a while. As we've said, anything even remotely connected with either pregnancy or babies is bound to trigger painful feelings. This may cause otherwise dauntless souls to avoid supermarkets, department stores, parks, or wherever mothers and babies are likely to be. Baby showers, christenings, or first birthday parties are sure-fire reminders. "Don't go to baby showers and pretend to enjoy it — you torture yourself and embarrass others," advises a woman who lost her baby in her eighth month.

Although you can't avoid all uncomfortable situations it is often possible to avoid those that you can anticipate will be painful. Alternatively, some women believe that facing those things that make them uncomfortable is necessary and even hastens the healing process.

Expect to feel waves of sadness return when you visit your obstetrician's office for a postpartum checkup. This was the place where you went in happier times, and also, perhaps, where you learned the bad news. Several women reported that their postpartum visit to the obstetrician's office was very upsetting, and, as one said, "I absolutely hated sitting around the sitting room at my checkup, with all those pregnant women. I don't know how else this could have been handled from the doctor's point of view, but it certainly was no fun sitting there, especially with all the baby care magazines all around."

Some women suggest calling ahead before the visit to request being seen on a day normally reserved for gynecology patients, or requesting the first appointment in a session so as not to have to sit in a waiting room filled with pregnant women. Another suggestion is to inform office nurses and staff of the loss so as to avoid uncomfortable questions about how the baby is doing. If at all possible, have your husband accompany you for your first postpartum visit. He will want to hear what the doctor has to say and he will probably have questions he would like answered. Further, he can be a source of support to you during this predictably difficult time. Think about taking along a close friend or a family member if your spouse is not available.

It is important that you discuss all of your questions and all of your concerns with your physician. Although you may be tempted to avoid sharing your feelings about or toward him or her, it is often helpful to do so. You may feel that he could have done more, that he made a mistake, that he should have been more supportive, or that he did all that he could, but that you let him down. Also, let him know how you are doing emotionally so that he can assess whether counseling or joining a support group might be helpful to you.

One of the things that your physician may want to discuss with you is his or her understanding of what may have caused the loss. If fetal tissue was available for examination by a pathologist, a report of these findings will also be reviewed. Last, he will advise you about planning for future pregnancies. If he feels that it is important to do diagnostic tests or to initiate treatment of some sort before you try to conceive again, this, too, will be discussed.

Activity
Keeping busy is an excellent way to cope as long as you don't use it to avoid dealing with your feelings: "I have a neighbor and dear friend who is a psychiatric nurse. She encouraged me to come over and cry and talk a lot, which probably kept me from having a nervous breakdown or committing suicide. She talked me into getting a job — any job to keep me busy and put me back into the world again — gave me a purpose for getting dressed and looking good. I got a job as a saleslady in a dress store, and it helped. I cried terribly the days I didn't work. Work kept me together."

A second woman commented, "Keeping busy for a while really helped. I devised all sorts of projects. We took a trip. Ultimately, though, the only thing that really helped was facing up to my grief, my depression — sinking to the depths for me . . . and then deciding I was tired of being unhappy. It was time to get on with life. This took about ten months altogether."

Seeking Help
Normally grief gradually diminishes as time passes. When this does not occur you have reason to be concerned that mourning is not

progressing as it should. The persistence of denial, of symptoms of depression (sleep difficulty, loss of appetite, irritability, crying, fatigue) or of intense feelings of guilt, anger, blame, or worthlessness is an indication that you might be having difficulty resolving your grief. Another is the persistence of psychosomatic symptoms (headache, unexplained pain, stomach upset, to name a few) or of self-destructive thoughts or behavior.

Most women find that the loss of a pregnancy or the death of a child is one of life's most agonizing experiences. You are not a failure if you have difficulty coping with the pain. If the pain feels unbearable, or if any of the warning signs just mentioned are present, you should consider seeking help. Increasingly, both professionals and women's support groups are becoming aware that women who have lost a pregnancy or delivered a stillborn child need and deserve such help. Resources are available locally in many communities through clinics and support groups.

Many couples have found that it is very helpful to talk with others who have lost a pregnancy. Since they have been through a similar experience, they know what your loss has been like. They may be able to offer you advice, consolation, and needed support. "Talk to other people who have lost a baby — suddenly they are everywhere," says a young woman, Debbie. "Believe me, they'll more than balance all those 'Oh, don't worry, you'll have another' comments that you are bound to get. Let people know that you have lost something important. Don't keep it bottled up inside."

You might want to join a support group for parents like yourself, or you may even want to organize one. Those who have taken part in such groups claim that the experience of being in a group with people who intuitively know what they had been through was greatly beneficial to them. Among the benefits that membership offered were being able to learn firsthand about how others coped, sharing experiences and feelings, and being able to help others. (For support resources, see appendix.)

Individual psychotherapy or counseling is another route people take to help them cope with their grief. After losing her baby during labor, Christine offered this comment: "Counseling helped me see that my reaction to the death of the child I had envisioned so clearly was not abnormal or overly strong. The pain and shock I felt was normal and experienced by many."

Another woman described her experience: "In counseling I could look forward to releasing my feelings without bugging my friends and husband, all of whom were getting tired of the subject. I definitely got better during this period, but whether it was because of the counseling or because I'd hit rock bottom and was determined to get over my depression, I don't know. Probably some of each. The counseling did give me some insights into why this particular matter had hit me so hard when generally I cope well with problems. Those insights made me feel better about myself — they lessened my guilt about not coping better."

"Counseling showed me I was still a woman," Dorothy, a soft-spoken and attractive red-haired woman, said, "and no less of one because of being unable to have children. It made me look at myself through different eyes. I think counseling helped me to deal with the unexpected emptiness."

How do you decide if you need counseling? Ask yourself if you are able to cope with your emotions. You may need counseling if you have overwhelming feelings of depression, anger or hopelessness, or are feeling so incapacitated by your feelings that you are unable to function.

Planning Another Pregnancy

One way of resolving your loss is by planning for future parenthood, either by trying to get pregnant again or by pursuing adoption.

Before trying to conceive again, you should discuss with your doctor what would be a reasonable waiting period. Your body and your emotions need time to recover. Pregnancy is stressful: another pregnancy may raise hopes, anxieties, and tensions before you are ready to deal with them.

You may want to meet with your physician to discuss the cause of death and to obtain a prognosis for future pregnancies. If you were dissatisfied with any aspect of the care you received, talk over your grievances with your doctor. If they can't be resolved, consider changing physicians.

"Find the best medical specialist you can — one who treats you like a human being," a social worker suggested. "I did, and it made all the difference in the world. I had total confidence in my doctor and felt like he really cared for me as a person. That meant a great deal to me."

Those who have experienced the loss of more than one pregnancy or have a history of infertility might consider consulting with an infertility specialist and/or a specialist in high-risk pregnancy.

SUMMARY

It is likely that your life has been significantly altered both by the pregnancy and by the loss you have experienced. Losing a baby may have been your first confrontation with death, your first realization that some events in life are out of your control. Feelings of depression, anxiety, and hopelessness arise not only from the immediate loss, but from an awareness that nothing in life is certain.

This view was expressed by a woman named Janet: "My miscarriage and infertility problems had a great effect on me. While it was a very difficult time, I believe I learned a great deal about myself and about other people. I also learned how important family and children are to me. I learned that I could not cope well with all crises. Previous to this I had always assumed I could handle whatever came my way. I am a deeper, more thoughtful, and more sympathetic person than before. I did not dislike myself before, but I like the 'new me' better. I also fully understand that events in life control us to a far greater extent than I had previously realized. I am more prepared for what life may now deal me. I realize I cannot totally control my destiny."

Grief is a painful fact of life. Fully experienced, it offers one the opportunity to expand one's consciousness, to grow, and to share with family and friends. Stoicism may be greatly admired by some, but only by grappling with grief can one eventually be free of it.

Normally grief gradually diminishes as time passes. However, even when it seems as if the worst pain is finally over, you may find that, on occasion, you still experience periods of sadness, distress, and yearning. Sometimes these feelings appear to rise out of the blue: sometimes they are triggered by some painful reminder. As with any loss, even years later you will feel some pain when you remember your loss. The anniversary of your child's death, encounters with children born at about the time that your child would have been: all can reawaken the pain.

It is important to remember that one does not easily get over a loss of the dimension that you have experienced. Mourning takes time. There is no one cure for the pain you feel. Even if you conceive and deliver a healthy baby, it will not erase the loss from your mind. Although the pain diminishes, there will always be reminders, and there will always be the loss of what could have been.

II

Types of Loss ❧ ❧ ❧ ❧

2

Miscarriage —
An Unrecognized Loss

Susan, a thirty-year-old teacher, and Mike, three years older, were elated when a test showed that Susan was pregnant after six months of trying to conceive. Ten days after the test, Susan began spotting and called her physician. After a pelvic examination, the doctor advised: "Take it easy and let's wait and see. You can continue with your normal routine, but rest as much as you can." For two weeks, she worked only part-time, living in dread that she would lose the baby they wanted so much. Their hopes and excitement over the pregnancy turned to worry when, one evening, the bleeding changed to a red, heavy flow and Susan began to experience intense pelvic pain. Mike rushed her to the emergency room of a hospital, to be met there by her doctor. An hour later, she delivered fetal tissue. Her doctor scheduled a D and C (dilation and curettage) for the next morning to remove from the uterus anything of the pregnancy tissue that might remain. Susan and Mike were shocked at the terrible physical and emotional trauma they had been through during those three weeks. They asked themselves: "How could this happen to two healthy people? What went wrong?"

Although most women know other women who have miscarried, few tend to think about it very much until it happens to them. Susan later reflected: "I now know that miscarriage is fairly common and that it can happen to anyone. Why hadn't I ever heard of it happening to anyone until my miscarriage?"

Because the infant death rate is low in the United States, it is common for couples to interpret a positive pregnancy test as a virtual guarantee that they will have a baby at the end of nine months. Susan said: "I suspect if I'd heard more about miscarriage when I was growing up, it might be easier to deal with, but my whole impression was a pregnancy equals a baby, which just isn't so for some of us."

Miscarriage is defined as the spontaneous or natural termination of a pregnancy prior to the twentieth week of gestation. Most couples who have experienced a miscarriage (or spontaneous abortion, as it is also called) are surprised to learn that it is not an unusual event. Few are aware that at least one in five pregnancies ends this way. In fact, the real incidence of miscarriage is even higher than these figures indicate, because statistics do not record those recognized miscarriages that do not come to a physician's attention, or those that go unrecognized and are noted only as delayed or unusually heavy menstrual periods.

With at least a 20 percent chance of miscarriage, why aren't couples aware of this possibility? For one thing, many doctors do not discuss the risk of miscarriage with their obstetric patients. When asked why not, they answer with some variation on "Most pregnancies turn out well, so why should I interfere with my patients' happiness and cause them to worry about something that probably won't happen?" This response indicates that even physicians, aware of the statistical risk of miscarriage, experience difficulty acknowledging that pregnancy sometimes ends in death rather than life. When miscarriage does occur, most couples are totally unprepared. They think of it as the kind of thing that just doesn't happen.

WARNING SIGNS

Women who miscarry usually have some previous warning. Depending on how advanced the pregnancy is, there are a number of signs and symptoms: vaginal bleeding, pelvic pain, no longer "feeling pregnant," and cessation of fetal movement or heartbeat. A fairly typical miscarriage begins with dark brown or red staining lasting several days, which may be accompanied by low abdominal pain and/or backache. This is followed by cramplike abdominal pain and heavy bleeding, and eventually by the passage of fetal and placental tissue.

Vaginal Bleeding

About 20 percent of pregnant women experience vaginal bleeding during the first twenty weeks of pregnancy. Half of these pregnancies will terminate in miscarriage, while the others will reach term successfully. Since it is initially impossible to determine when bleeding will result in miscarriage, most physicians consider any bleeding in early pregnancy a sign of "threatened abortion" or miscarriage.

A doctor should be consulted whenever vaginal bleeding occurs during pregnancy. The seepage may be dark brown, which indicates old blood, or bright red, a sign of more active bleeding. Often the doctor will recommend a pelvic examination to determine if the cervix is closed (an indication that active labor has not begun). He will also try to find the cause of the bleeding. Besides a threatened miscarriage, other causes of vaginal bleeding include ectopic pregnancy, cervical erosions and polyps, and implantation bleeding.

If bleeding is slight or short-lived, the physician probably would decide to wait and see before ordering diagnostic tests. However, persistent bleeding usually warrants a more thorough assessment of the situation.

Pelvic Pain

Cramplike low abdominal pain usually accompanies the bleeding and increases in intensity as the process continues. If a pelvic examination is carried out at this time, it will reveal that the cervix has begun to shorten and dilate, forewarning in most cases the beginning of labor and the inevitability of miscarriage.

Absence or Disappearance of Signs and Symptoms of Pregnancy

Many women experience symptoms such as morning sickness, fatigue, and breast engorgement during the first trimester. A number of women who miscarry either fail to have such symptoms of pregnancy at all or, having had them, notice that they have stopped. In the latter case, bleeding commonly starts several days later.

For some women, the onset of miscarriage is heralded by a vague sense that something is wrong. It is not uncommon for a woman to feel less pregnant and wonder if her breasts are less full, if her abdomen looks less protuberant, or if her queasiness and fatigue have suddenly decreased. These physical sensations can be accompanied by a strange kind of tension, as well as by feelings of dread.

Depending on what warning signs are present, the outcome of the pregnancy may either be known immediately or unclear for a while, at least. The eventual outcome may be unclear when such symptoms as vaginal bleeding, pelvic heaviness, or an apparent decrease in nausea, breast engorgement, or fatigue are present. The symptoms of a threatened miscarriage can persist for anywhere from a few hours to days, weeks, or even months before they cease or miscarriage occurs.

The absence of a previously present heartbeat is an absolute sign of fetal death. Likewise, if the woman's subjective sense that fetal movement has ceased for more than twenty-four hours is confirmed by the examining physician, fetal death may be diagnosed soon after the first warning signs are noted.

Sometimes it is possible to determine the probable outcome of a "threatened miscarriage" using a variety of diagnostic tests. When a woman conceives, a hormone, human chorionic gonadotropin (HCG), produced by the fetal trophoblast (the placenta) may be detected in the mother's urine or blood. Measurement of the beta subunit fraction of HCG can let your doctor know if the fetal placenta is still functioning and whether the fetus is still alive. (This is a more sensitive test than a routine pregnancy test.) Another procedure, the diagnostic ultrasound, is also used to assess whether the fetus appears to be viable. This test uses sound waves to form a picture, and in this way can demonstrate whether an embryonic sac and a fetus are present, indicating that the pregnancy is still viable. Likewise, if the pregnancy is sufficiently advanced for a fetal heartbeat to be present, ultrasound examination will reveal if one can be found, thereby determining whether the fetus is dead or alive.

COPING WITH THE SIGNS OF MISCARRIAGE

Women respond differently to the first signs of difficulty. Some feel an immediate sense of panic and dread, others feel concern but remain optimistic, and some feel shocked, disbelieving, and frozen. If the warning signs persist for a prolonged period of time, it is likely that periods of optimism will alternate with times of despair and disbelief. Susan, whose miscarriage was described earlier, tearfully described her feelings of cold dread as she saw that the paper with which she was wiping herself was stained with blood. "I just sat there not believing that this was happening to me. I think that I cried but I don't remember feeling very much. I know that for the next few hours I kept going back into the bathroom to see if there was still blood — each time wishing that it had all been a mistake. When I called my doctor and told him what had happened, he asked me to come over to his office so that he could examine me. I felt totally panicked. When he examined me and found that my cervix was closed and that my uterus seemed to be the right size, I felt a bit relieved, maybe it was not going to be so bad after all. I can hardly remember anything about the next two weeks other than checking to see if I was still bleeding — feeling hopeful when I wasn't, and terror-stricken when I was."

In some ways the most difficult period begins with the first awareness that there may be something wrong. There can be days, weeks, or even months of uncertainty. Reactions to this situation vary. It is not uncommon for a woman to put her feelings about the pregnancy "on hold" as a way of protecting herself against the possibility that it will be lost. Nor is it unusual for her to be anxious, obsessed, and incapable of thinking about anything else.

This period of uncertainty can be a difficult one. Nonetheless, many women feel best about themselves when they try to gain some control over the situation: for instance, informing the physician when any of the above "danger signs" are present. It is tempting to deny the implications of what may be happening — to tell yourself that you are just imagining it. Many women who did told us they remember thinking at the time, "I don't want to disturb my doctor"; "I'm just overreacting — I'll feel like a fool if everything is normal"; and "It's just minor. I'll wait to see what happens." But denying the problem or acting stoically isn't a good idea. Being afraid of bad news is all the more reason to take action, so you can either relax or begin to deal with what may occur. It is better to make a mistake because you're too concerned; waiting too long to seek medical attention can jeopardize the pregnancy, your health, or even your life.

Your physician probably will take your concerns seriously and tell you his initial impression as well as what course of action he plans to follow for the present, or anticipates following in the future if your symptoms either continue as they are or became more severe.

Women who experienced a miscarriage have told us how important the support of husband, family, and friends was to them. Many found it helpful to share fears and concerns, to have someone accompany them to the doctor's office or to the hospital for diagnostic tests, and to receive help in making whatever decisions needed to be made. Generally it was agreed that the concern and caring of others were helpful in getting them through this very stressful and alarming time.

THE PHYSICAL EXPERIENCE OF MISCARRIAGE

For many women the physical experience of miscarriage is upsetting, even extremely frightening. Often one is unprepared for what an actual miscarriage is apt to be like. In addition, since miscarriage occurs early in pregnancy, most women will not yet have had any formal preparation for labor and delivery. Very early miscarriage may be quite similar to a very heavy menstrual period. In contrast, late miscarriage may follow a course not unlike that of a full-term labor and delivery.

It is important to know that heavy bleeding, with or without the passage of clots or tissue, is an indication of impending miscarriage. Cramping or low abdominal pain and watery discharge from the amniotic sac through the vagina are other common indications.

Sometimes miscarriage follows such a rapid course that it is not possible to get to the doctor's office or to a hospital in time. If this should happen to you, you should, if possible, place fetal tissue, which appears as a grayish red mass or blood clot, in a clean container and bring it along to the hospital for the pathologist to examine.

If the miscarriage occurs while you are in the hospital, the physician will check to see if all of the pregnancy tissue (fetus, placenta, and amniotic sac) have been passed. If it happens at home, he or she will conduct an exam afterward.

If all of the fetal and placental tissue has been expelled, the miscarriage is considered to have been complete. Pain and severe bleeding stop, and usually no further treatment is necessary. However, a blood-stained vaginal discharge, called lochia, may persist for several days, until the site where the fertilized egg had implanted itself in the uterus has healed. "Complete" miscarriage usually occurs before the eighth week of pregnancy and is uncommon later in pregnancy.

When only part of the pregnancy tissue is expelled, the miscarriage is said to be "incomplete." Incomplete miscarriages happen more frequently after the eighth week of pregnancy, after the placenta is more strongly attached to the uterus.

If the physician is not sure if the miscarriage was complete, he will perform a minor operation known as a D and C (see page 29) to empty your uterus. During a D and C, the cervix is stretched and a spoon-shaped instrument called a curette is inserted through the cervix and used to scrape the uterus. The procedure is usually performed under anesthesia and in a hospital.

Immediately after spontaneous miscarriage or after a D and C, the uterine muscles contract. This action blocks exposed uterine blood vessels, keeping bleeding to a minimum. When this happens, you may experience abdominal cramps much like menstrual cramps or labor pains. These cramps, or afterpains, are usually most intense right after the delivery of the fetus has occurred. Thereafter, they decrease in intensity and frequency. Some women have afterpains for a day or two following the loss of a pregnancy.

Many women who have had a second-trimester miscarriage have found that on the second to fourth day afterward their breasts became engorged with milk. Since one's body has no way of knowing that the fetus has died, it reflexively prepares for breast feeding. Engorgement may cause some physical discomfort, but normally the actual physical pain is less troublesome than the emotional pain that may accompany it. Usually, engorgement will diminish in a day or two. It is important to refrain from expressing milk to alleviate discomfort, as doing this only leads to an increase in milk production. Aspirin may be taken if there is a great deal of pain. Hot wet compresses or ice packs applied to the breasts can also be used to decrease discomfort.

MISSED ABORTION

Sometimes the fetus dies but is not expelled. This type of miscarriage is classified as a missed abortion. A missed abortion may occur at any time during the first twenty weeks of pregnancy. Typically, a woman who has a missed abortion has experienced several months of normal pregnancy, with fatigue, enlargement of the uterus, breast fullness, and possible nausea. After the fetus dies, the signs of pregnancy gradually disappear. Commonly, the woman will notice that her breasts are less full, that she no longer experiences nausea, and that she has lost some weight. A brownish vaginal discharge is usually observed, and in more advanced pregnancies fetal movements are no longer felt. Pelvic examination will reveal that not only has the uterus failed to grow, but it has become smaller and lacks the soft consistency characteristic of pregnancy. Some women with a missed abortion will not have any vaginal discharge or bleeding. Then the presumptive diagnosis is usually based on the absence of normal uterine growth.

If a missed abortion is suspected, the diagnosis of fetal death can be established through testing. Within several days of the death, placental function usually ceases and human chorionic gonadotropin (HCG) is no longer produced. Urine or blood tests for the level of HCG often read negative (no HCG present) soon after the fetus dies; thus, if a previously positive test becomes negative, it is likely that fetal death has occurred. Sometimes, however, the placenta continues to function for several weeks and the test remains positive. In such cases, ultrasonic examination can demonstrate whether or not the amniotic (fetal) sac is empty, which indicates that no fetus can be detected, or whether a fetal heartbeat is no longer present.

Labor: Spontaneous or Induced?
Once the diagnosis of fetal death is made, there are two possible courses of action: awaiting spontaneous labor, which usually occurs within a few weeks, or having labor induced.

The advantage of waiting until labor begins spontaneously is that one avoids the risk that the cervix will be damaged by forceful dilation. However, since a potentially life-threatening problem, intravascular coagulation (clotting), can occur when a dead fetus is carried by the mother for more than four weeks after fetal death has occurred, most physicians will allow the pregnancy to be carried no longer than this before suggesting that labor be induced.

Still, some women prefer not to have labor induced immediately. Some who have made this choice have felt that they needed a little time with their baby before they were willing to let it go. Others expressed a need for time to deal with the death, while a number of women preferred that labor and delivery be as natural as possible.

Many women, on the other hand, find that it is very upsetting to carry a dead fetus. Instead, they elect to have labor artificially induced. For those who have suffered through days or weeks of threatened miscarriage and subsequent fetal death, the decision to have labor induced is a means "to get it over with and go on with life," as one woman put it.

Recently, the use of prostaglandins has made the induction of labor in a woman with a missed abortion safe and reliable.

Georgia and Tom chose to wait for labor to begin naturally after they learned of their baby's death at five months. "We had been reading about natural childbirth and had just begun attending classes in it. We wanted to quickly finish learning about it and continue as we had planned. We felt it would give us some time to adjust to the death. We couldn't believe it at first. And we knew we wanted to try again and the labor and delivery experience would be helpful in a future pregnancy."

The physician usually discusses the pros and cons of both options. However, unless there are overriding medical considerations, the final choice is usually left to the woman.

It is common to feel a resurgence of grief once delivery has taken place, even if mourning took place when fetal death was first diagnosed. This is because at the delivery, secret hopes that the fetus "was really alive in spite of all indications to the contrary" must be finally abandoned.

THE HOSPITAL STAY

If miscarriage occurs prior to the twentieth week of pregnancy and all pregnancy tissue is passed spontaneously, hospitalization may not be necessary. However, if fetal death occurs after the twentieth week, if the miscarriage is incomplete, or if it is not possible to determine whether or not all tissue has been passed, the woman will be admitted to the hospital so that a D and C can be performed. A   D and C is done whenever there is a danger that the miscarriage may have been "incomplete," since the failure to remove all pregnancy tissue from the uterus may cause hemorrhage.

Many factors conspire to make the hospital experience a difficult one for the woman who has miscarried. Since the routines in most hospitals are planned around women delivering healthy full-term babies, it is quite likely that many hospital practices and regulations do not meet the miscarrying woman's needs.

Hospitals differ greatly in their treatment of women who have miscarried. The best ones offer a choice of accommodations, helpful and supportive nursing care, and even in-hospital counseling. However, such is not always the case.

Women who were hospitalized told us that the experience was less painful than it might have otherwise been when they were able to arrange the following things:

(1) to have their husbands be with them as much as possible, including during labor, and delivery and in the recovery room; when overnight hospitalization was necessary, some women asked that their husbands be allowed to stay with them;

(2) to be hospitalized on a floor other than the maternity floor;

(3) to have a private, rather than a shared, room if desired;

(4) to discuss in advance with the physician whether to have local or general anesthesia during delivery or during the D and C;

(5) to decide in advance whether or not to see the fetus;

(6) to decide how the fetal tissue would be disposed of.

(Since hospitalization is an integral part of the stillbirth experience, it is covered in more detail on pages 64–67.)

CAUSES

One of the first questions couples ask after a miscarriage is "What caused the miscarriage to occur?" In many cases, unfortunately, it is not possible for the physician to determine the specific cause, even following pathological examination of fetal tissue. Sometimes it is impossible to determine whether or not there are any abnormalities present. In other situations, one or more potential causes may be found but it is not possible to determine whether one particular factor is, in fact, the significant one. This means that it is quite likely that you will not be able to find out exactly what caused you to miscarry. This is frustrating in and of itself, but doubly troubling in that the failure to determine a cause leaves both you and your physician in the dark about what to look for and what treatments to try in subsequent pregnancies. Reflecting on two miscarriages, Lynn said: "I wish someone could diagnose the *why* of either miscarriage. The worst part is having to go through all that without anyone ever being able to give an explanation."

Abnormal Fetal Development

Medical research has demonstrated that the single most common cause of miscarriage is an abnormality in the development of the embryo, fetus, or placenta that is incompatible with life. A pregnancy is destined to fail from the very outset if the chromosomal or genetic abnormality is too severe to permit the fertilized ovum to survive. When the embryo dies, hormonal support for the pregnancy stops. Sometime after this, the defective embryo is expelled. Since the developmental abnormality in these "blighted" ova is so severe that survival is not possible, there is no treatment that can save the pregnancy.

Most blighted ova pregnancies result from random factors that are unlikely to be repeated and so do not pose a risk to subsequent pregnancies or to future children: 50 to 60 percent of early spontaneous abortions are associated with chromosomal abnormalities. In most of these instances the parents' chromosomes are normal, and a new mutation is responsible for the chromosomal abnormality. The earlier the miscarriage, the more likely it is that chromosomal factors are responsible.

In accepting her loss, one woman expressed it this way: "I deeply feel that if a miscarriage occurs, there is a reason and it's best to let it go. The baby would have had problems and it's nature's sad but wise way of protecting everyone concerned."

Hormonal Factors

(1) PROGESTERONE It is well known that the reproductive hormones estrogen and progesterone play an active role both in permitting pregnancy to occur and in maintaining pregnancy once conception takes place. What is less well established, however, is what role, if any, progesterone deficiency plays in causing miscarriage.

Research is currently under way studying the effects of progesterone deficiency on the uterine lining (the endometrium) during the postovulatory phase of the menstrual cycle. Investigators have attempted to treat women with an inadequate postovulatory phase (believed to be caused by progesterone deficiency) with progesterone prior to implantation of the fertilized ovum in the hope that miscarriage will be prevented.

Another research project focuses on giving progesterone to women with a well-established pregnancy. These women were considered at risk because of existing symptoms of "threatened miscarriage" or a previous history of pregnancy loss. This treatment was based on the theory that either the placenta or the corpus luteum might not be producing adequate amounts of progesterone and that the administration of progesterone may be effective in preventing miscarriage.

Unfortunately, to date, neither type of treatment has been definitively demonstrated to be effective. In addition, there is evidence that prenatal exposure to female sex hormones may cause developmental abnormalities in the fetus. For these reasons, most physicians are reluctant to prescribe progesterone for the prevention of miscarriage unless a postovulatory-phase defect can be clearly demonstrated and all other types of treatment have been exhausted.

(2) ENDOCRINE SECRETIONS There is some evidence that disorders of the thyroid or the pituitary gland may in a very few women interfere with their ability to become pregnant and, once they are pregnant, may increase the risk of miscarrying.

Uterine Disorders

Some uterine abnormalities may affect the growth and development of the fetus. A woman may be born with two uterine compartments instead of the usual single chamber. Others may have either an unusually small uterus, or other developmental abnormalities. The presence of one or more large uterine fibroid tumors (benign growths) may also pose a problem.

While both uterine abnormalities and fibroid tumors are associated with an increased risk of miscarriage, not every woman who has these conditions experiences difficulty in carrying a pregnancy to term. If, however, the specific uterine abnormality is such that the fetus does not have room to grow, miscarriage will eventually occur. Surgical correction of uterine structural problems and fibroids offers many women with these problems a good chance for success in subsequent pregnancies.

Cervical Incompetence

An "incompetent" cervix, a cervix that fails to remain closed for the duration of the pregnancy, is still another structural abnormality that may be associated with an increased risk of miscarriage. Why some women have cervical incompetence is not known. In others, it seems to occur secondary to cervical damage sustained during dilation of the cervix for tests, or in the course of traumatic delivery or therapeutic abortion. Characteristically, the woman with an incompetent cervix usually does well during the first trimester of pregnancy. But as the fetus increases in size and weight during the second trimester, the already weakened cervix dilates prematurely, thus threatening the continuation of the pregnancy. Since this dilation occurs in the absence of painful uterine contractions, it often goes unrecognized by the woman and undiagnosed by the physician until the pregnancy is already lost. When diagnosed early, on the other hand, it can be treated by encircling the cervix with stitches or with a band that keeps it closed. This procedure is most often performed some time between the fourteenth and twentieth week of pregnancy. The closure is usually removed by cutting the band or the stitches when it is time for labor.

Cervical incompetence is a relatively rare cause of miscarriage. Only approximately one in a hundred miscarriages occur for this reason. However, it should be considered as a possible cause of miscarriage when the pregnancy is lost between the third and the sixth month. Moreover, women who have had one late miscarriage should be followed closely in subsequent pregnancies for signs of cervical incompetence.

Other Factors That May Cause Miscarriage

(1) BLOOD TYPE INCOMPATIBILITY Controversy exists about whether blood type incompatibility of either the Rh or ABO system in the parents increases the likelihood that early miscarriage will occur. Blood group incompatibility, however, has clearly been demonstrated to contribute to the loss of pregnancy after twenty weeks.

(2) DES EXPOSURE Diethylstilbestrol (DES), a synthetic estrogen, was first used as a medication to prevent fetal loss in 1945. It was used for this purpose until 1971, when an association was discovered between DES exposure and a rare form of vaginal cancer in the daughters of women so treated. There followed shortly the discovery that DES exposure was also associated with unusual but characteristic abnormalities of the vagina and cervix among these daughters. Although it was originally feared that these vaginal and cervical abnormalities might be associated with the later development of vaginal cancer, this concern appears not to have been borne out. Happily, the overall incidence of vaginal cancer in DES daughters is also much lower than was originally predicted.

In recent years, DES exposure has been linked to a variety of fertility problems. Clinical studies have indicated that women whose mothers took DES show a somewhat reduced ability to conceive, compared to the overall population. DES exposure has also been held responsible for a higher than usual incidence of tubal pregnancy. Although as yet the association between DES exposure and both miscarriage and prematurity has not been conclusively established, there is evidence to indicate that women exposed to DES have a higher than average incidence of uterine abnormalities, cervical incompetence, first and second trimester miscarriage, and premature births.

(3) MATERNAL DISEASE An increased rate of fetal loss (miscarriage and stillbirth) has been linked with a number of infectious diseases.

Some viral agents are thought to be responsible for both congenital malformations and miscarriage. A higher than normal incidence of both types of difficulty are found in women infected with the following viruses: rubella (German measles), cytomegalovirus, herpes simplex virus, measles, mumps, polio, chicken pox, and hepatitis. Fortunately, these infections tend to be quite uncommon during pregnancy.

T mycoplasma, an infectious agent which has characteristics of both bacteria and viruses, has been found in the tissues of some aborted fetuses. This microorganism has been implicated as a cause of both infertility and miscarriage. Although there is no definite evidence that T mycoplasma causes infertility or miscarriage, many physicians treat couples with a course of antibiotics (usually tetracycline) if either member has a positive culture.

The risk of miscarrying is somewhat increased for women who have certain chronic illnesses. This is particularly true when the illness is severe. Diabetes, systemic lupus erythematosis, some heart conditions, kidney disease, and markedly elevated blood pressure, are all associated with an increased rate of miscarriage.

(4) RADIATION EXPOSURE Exposure to significant amounts of ionizing radiation has been linked with both an increased incidence of miscarriage and an increased incidence of congenital malformations. Exposure to all types of X rays should be avoided during pregnancy unless absolutely necessary. If at all possible, ultrasound, which uses high-frequency sound waves, should be used in preference to diagnostic X rays during pregnancy.

(5) MALNUTRITION While poor nutrition has been implicated in many complications of pregnancy, only very severe malnutrition predisposes to an increased incidence of early pregnancy loss.

(6) MATERNAL AGE The risk of fetal loss of all types, including miscarriage, is significantly greater for women under the age of twenty and over thirty-five than for women between these ages. Why this is so is not known.

(7) USE OF ALCOHOL The Surgeon General's Advisory on Alcohol and Pregnancy warns that alcohol consumption during pregnancy,

especially during the early months, has been demonstrated to be harmful to the fetus. An increase in the rate of miscarriage is one of several hazards associated with alcohol use during pregnancy. Women who consume one ounce of absolute alcohol (two standard drinks) twice a week have been reported to experience a significantly increased rate of miscarriage. The effect of lower levels of alcohol consumption or less frequent use carries an as yet unknown risk, as no absolutely safe level of alcohol consumption has been established.

(8) USE OF MARIJUANA The American Medical Association has officially labeled marijuana a dangerous drug. Marijuana use has been demonstrated to affect reproductive function adversely in a variety of ways, including increasing the likelihood that miscarriage will occur. In a study in which female monkeys were treated with THC, the active chemical in marijuana, for three to five years at doses comparable to daily consumption for humans, the miscarriage rate was found to increase significantly.

(9) USE OF TOBACCO Smoking has been implicated in increasing the risk of miscarriage. Although all of the evidence is not yet in, it seems advisable that cigarette smoking should be stopped during pregnancy.

(10) USE OF CAFFEINE There is evidence to indicate that the consumption of caffeine during pregnancy is associated with an increase in the incidence of miscarriage. It is advised that beverages such as coffee, tea, and colas and drugs containing caffeine be eliminated from use during pregnancy.

(11) TRAUMA Only in extremely rare instances are either physical or emotional traumas thought to be responsible for causing miscarriage. Travel by car, train, or plane has not been associated with an increased incidence of miscarriage. Similarly, most pregnant women can work, exercise in moderation, and engage in sexual intercourse without jeopardy either to themselves or to the fetus. The reason for this is that the fetus is well protected. First, it is surrounded by a pool of amniotic fluid, which acts as a shock absorber, then by the

membraneous amniotic sac, and by the muscular wall of the uterus. The mother's visceral organs and, finally, her skin form additional layers of protection. Pregnancy has been known to continue successfully despite serious accidents, major surgery, exhaustion, or emotional stress. In fact, it is doubtful whether anything but the most extreme environmental factors can disrupt a well-established pregnancy.

(12) ENVIRONMENTAL FACTORS Exposure to pesticides and other toxic chemicals should be avoided during pregnancy, as evidence is accumulating to indicate the harmful effect of many of these substances on the developing fetus.

Psychological Factors

When a woman miscarries, she, her husband, family, and physician all seek a tangible reason for why the pregnancy failed. Frequently, none is found. Most couples have a great deal of difficulty dealing with this uncertainty. Every event or occurrence is scrutinized in an attempt to find an explanation for the unexplainable. It is almost as if a "cause" must be found before the miscarriage can be put behind them.

An entire mythology about miscarriage has developed over the years and attests to the strong need to understand what has happened. Most myths imply that a particular activity, event, or psychological experience, one that is deemed of marginal acceptability during pregnancy, is responsible for the miscarriage.

The notion found in traditional psychoanalytic theory that miscarriage may be caused by emotional conflicts is one such myth. Classical theory maintains that miscarriage may be a physical expression of the mother's negative or ambivalent feelings toward either the pregnancy or the mothering role. This theory offers little support to the woman who has miscarried and, in fact, quite clearly blames the victim for bringing her difficulties upon herself.

The research studies and clinical treatment upon which this theory was based were both seriously flawed. It is unfortunate that until the past few years, these flaws were totally overlooked and thus a theory that was decidedly hostile to women was accepted by both the medical establishment and society.

The psychosomatic theory of miscarriage was based upon the clinical studies and treatment of women who had previously experienced one or more miscarriages. According to the investigators, these women were more immature, emotional, and "neurotic" than other women. However, the investigators failed to take into account what these women were like before they had miscarried, since they saw them only after the miscarriage. Most individuals experience the loss of a desired pregnancy as traumatic and have a period of heightened emotionality lasting anywhere from a week or so to several months afterward, so it is not unusual that researchers found the women to be "emotional." There is no real evidence that a woman's emotional state during the pregnancy influences whether or not she will miscarry, or that her emotional state afterward indicates anything meaningful about her emotional state before the loss of the pregnancy.

The utility of psychotherapeutic treatment in reversing a woman's tendency to repeatedly miscarry has been claimed but never actually demonstrated. Nevertheless, the alleged success of this treatment was used by supporters of the psychosomatic theory as evidence supporting their original claims. In sum, there is no solid evidence that supports the notion that emotional factors play a significant role in the causation of miscarriage.

WILL IT EVER HAPPEN AGAIN?

A concern commonly voiced by couples who have suffered a miscarriage is "What are the chances that our next pregnancy will be successful?" If the miscarriage was your first or second, the response to this question is quite encouraging. After one miscarriage, the statistical risk of having a second miscarriage is about the same as the risk of a miscarriage in the first place. In all likelihood, each was caused by random, unrelated events that have little likelihood of recurring.

A woman is said to be a "habitual aborter" if she has had three or more consecutive pregnancies terminating in miscarriage. Whether each of the miscarriages was caused by random factors, or whether they were caused by a recurrent, underlying difficulty must be assessed for each individual. Habitual abortion will be dealt with more extensively in the chapter "Multiple Losses."

TRYING AGAIN

There is some disagreement among physicians about how long to wait after a miscarriage before trying to conceive again. Ninety percent of women will have their first menstrual period four to six weeks after miscarrying. Some physicians feel that if a woman is anxious to conceive, she can begin trying after her first menstrual period. The more usual view is that the chance of a repeat miscarriage is decreased if she waits until she has had three normal periods before attempting a new pregnancy.

Sexual relations may be resumed when the bleeding has stopped and the cervix is closed, which usually occurs three to four weeks following a miscarriage.

Medical Treatment

Most cases of miscarriage have no discernible cause. The failure to find a cause is usually a good sign, as it indicates that random factors were probably responsible, and that a recurrent difficulty is not present.

Most physicians feel that it is unjustified to perform a comprehensive evaluation after a woman has had one miscarriage, because the odds are in favor of a nonspecific or random cause. Medical evaluation is usually recommended after a woman has miscarried two or three times consecutively. If evaluation reveals a specific cause, treatment will be aimed at dealing with that difficulty.

HORMONAL TREATMENT It is felt to be unjustified as a way of treating miscarriage of unknown cause. Estimates are that progesterone deficiency is involved in only 4 percent of miscarriages. In those cases where it can be demonstrated that the woman has a clear postovulatory-phase insufficiency due to progesterone deficiency, progesterone may be administered during the second phase of the cycle and during early pregnancy. There is no evidence that progesterone is effective in treating "threatened miscarriage" because by the time bleeding has started the pregnancy is usually unsalvage-able. Fetal death usually precedes the onset of bleeding by several days or weeks. Since this treatment may carry some potential risk to the fetus, it must always be carefully considered.

CHROMOSOMAL ABNORMALITIES These are found in a large percent-age of miscarried fetuses. The vast majority are probably caused by random, nonrepeatable mutations. Chromosomal study is usually recommended after the miscarriage of two, or more usually three, consecutive pregnancies. If a chromosomal abnormality is found that has a high likelihood of recurring in subsequent pregnancies, genetic counseling is normally suggested.

UTERINE ABNORMALITIES Uterine abnormalities may be diagnosed using a combination of pelvic examination and hysterogram (dye is inserted into the uterus and visualized by X ray). Surgical correction is performed whenever it increases the chance for a successful preg-nancy. Conditions that may be corrected surgically in many cases include uterine fibroid tumors, double uterus, and cervical weak-ness or incompetence.

Screening for Underlying Difficulties
Screening for systemic disease and thyroid gland malfunction may be attempted as part of a complete evaluation, although the likeli-hood of such screening being fruitful in an otherwise healthy, asymptomatic woman is very small.

One Woman's Story

MARCH 1979
I was unprepared for the unrelenting grief, for the intensity of it. I kept thinking, "What is wrong with me? I should be over this by now. I shouldn't be so obsessed with it all — the maternity shops I go by, the Pampers com-

mercials on television. I should be able to call my pregnant and recently delivered friends without struggling to carefully modulate my voice; without needing to give myself a pep talk before I dial the phone. And yet, I still cry. I cry out of control. I cry over trivia, and over everyday occurrences, and over how alone I feel. I still cling desperately to the hope that THIS month, I will be pregnant again, and be able to feel my belly growing and my breasts filling, and my baby kicking inside. My usual methods for coping with stress have been pretty useless."

I am a psychiatrist, and this somehow made me think that I would be able to handle my feelings rationally. I reasoned that many women go through things like this; I have close friends who have miscarried and I have other friends who have had trouble conceiving. I tell myself that I should be able to get through this without falling apart.

What I have learned in a most painful way was that before this happened to me, I really had no idea of what my friends had to bear. I had been as insensitive and ignorant toward them as I now feel people are to me. It wasn't all my fault, of course. They hadn't really tried to talk with me about what they were going through.

I didn't know before it happened to me that I would begin to wonder if there was something wrong with me, that I couldn't do this natural, simple thing that all other women do, often without even wanting to. Everything was as usual in my life: my work, my son, my home, my husband . . . EVERYTHING . . . *except that every minute feels like a year to me, every day takes forever, and all I can think about is loss, death, and the damn calendar. Spring is here, and instead of feeling happy, I feel miserable. I thought I would be round and well on my way by now, and instead, my body in its smallness seems a perpetual rebuke and a reminder of what I don't have. For everyone else the winter happened and is over, while I feel suspended in time, waiting, counting until I can be pregnant again.*

When I happen, by chance, to see a pregnant woman on the street, I can't control my need to stare. I feel miserably torn between fascination, envy, and rage that it isn't me that is pregnant.

I just wasn't prepared for how awful I feel: the isolation, the gauze wrapping of depression. In contrast to my usual ability to be funny, light, and social, I am unable to be casual or light about anything. I am obsessed with worry that something may be wrong with me; that I will miscarry again; that I'll never have another child.

Sometimes it is comforting to be with my son. At other times I can't tolerate my love for him, because he reminds me of what I have lost. I don't know why but I worry about his health, my health, my husband's health. I feel a sense of urgency about having another child: I worry that there will be too much space between children, and I worry that I am getting old. I don't seem to be able to relax, and wait the required months before trying again.

My second miscarriage was at eleven weeks, and it took about nine days from the time I started with a bit of brownish discharge to the day I miscarried. I've read that most women don't allow themselves to acknowledge the possibility of miscarriage, and so if it happens, it comes as a complete shock. My experience was quite different in that I had misgivings about this pregnancy from the beginning. Perhaps this was because I had had a very early miscarriage four months before; perhaps because I had had a healthy term pregnancy and I knew what it felt like. In any case, I'd had cramps early in the pregnancy and had never felt very pregnant. No nausea, almost no fatigue, few of the subtle physical changes that I had experienced the first time. I found myself continually trying to explain these vague misgivings to my husband and to my obstetrician. I felt that I didn't want to invest too much or tell too many people.

In some ways I was not surprised when I began to have some spotting. I was, nevertheless, intensely upset. I hesitated before checking with my doctor lest he think I was being "hysterical" and "overreacting." I spent four days doing little other than noting every twinge, cramp, and bit of vaginal discharge. On the fifth day I woke up feeling different. Less pregnant, even, than I had felt before. My stomach felt a little bit shrunken, my breasts totally untender.

My husband tried to be reassuring, but his calmness left me feeling isolated. I went to work, not knowing what else to do, because it all seemed so subjective. I tried to go through the day as if everything was fine, but I knew that everything was all wrong.

As I left work that evening and walked to my car, it was snowing. I was concentrating on not moving too fast so I wouldn't have more spotting. I got home; we ate dinner. I stood up to take some dishes to the sink and felt uncomfortably bloated for a moment; then I felt a warm sticky trickle run down my legs, and I ran into the bathroom.

Although I felt a terrible rush of fear, I tried to stay calm, partly so as not to upset my son, and partly to delay the impact of what I knew had happened. Looking at the bright red blood as it flowed into the toilet, I felt surprised to feel all of the things that I had thought I wouldn't experience, because I was psychologically so "well prepared." But they were all there: grief, disappointment, anger, emptiness, isolation, and uncertainty about what to do next. I didn't cry right away. I held myself together beautifully until I had to tell the people I cared about — my husband, my child, my parents and my sister, and a few special friends. With them, I couldn't be brave.

The next four days were a nightmare; perhaps the hardest time in my life so far. The uncertainty was so terrible that it was almost a relief when the miscarriage finally happened. During those four days I realized that doctors have so little to offer — they can't tell you what will happen, if the bleeding means that you are having a miscarriage, if staying off your feet really helps — they just don't know. I went to the hospital, had a blood test to check my hormone level, saw my doctor, and went home to bed.

The lab wasn't sure the test results would be ready the next day, a Friday: I might have to wait until Monday. It's strange how all my energy came to be focused on the results of that blood test, even though I knew that it wouldn't tell us very much. I knew that if the hormone level was low, it was fairly certain that the pregnancy wouldn't last. If it was high, then maybe I was not having a miscarriage after all. I continued to bleed; by Monday, I would be able to tell them, and the blood test would be irrelevant. Nevertheless, I called the lab every fifteen minutes.

I went to work Friday afternoon because it was my first day on a new job, and I felt it important to be there, even if only for a few hours. My husband picked me up at my car and drove me to the building my office was in so I wouldn't have to walk the two blocks. Although there was no reason to think that walking would hurt, we didn't want to take the chance. I called the lab every time I had a free moment between clients. By 5:00, they thought they'd have a result for me before the weekend. It turned out to be OK, a reasonably high HCG, which cheered me up a great deal. However, in the next few days my optimism proved to be ill founded.

I stayed in bed until Sunday. By that time, I'd had some pretty severe cramping and I began to wish for some resolution. The intensity of my feelings was getting to be too much for me; the only escape was sleep.

I had several hours of labor Sunday night. It stopped and started again at four or five on Monday morning. By seven or so, I had passed some tissue, which I could not bring myself to save in a jar, although I knew I should. My doctor had asked that I save any solid fragments so that he could make a diagnosis of why the pregnancy failed. But the thought of my would-be child in a container was too upsetting. When I felt something coming, I ran to the toilet, looked quickly, and flushed it down. I still believe it was the only thing I could have done.

So we went empty-handed to the hospital, my husband calling to cancel his day, and me calling to cancel mine before we walked out the door. I called one or two of my closest friends to tell them what was going on, then we left off our son with his sitter, as though it were a normal day.

In truth, by this time, I felt almost euphoric. The uncertainty was finally over. I'd go to the hospital, have a nice, antiseptic, sleepy cleanout, wait the required months and have another pregnancy. I felt that the preceding week had been the worst of my life. Now it was over and I could once again take control of what was happening to me.

The D and C went well, and I was able to leave the hospital that evening. I took the next day off from work to get myself back together: I needed to adjust to not being pregnant anymore. I took a long, glorious walk that day. It was one of the really crisp, sunny days of January with a brilliant blue sky, preceding the mush and gloom of February and March in Boston. I reveled in being able to move without worrying about whether I was bleeding or not — it didn't matter anymore. In fact, the more I bled, the more I felt cleansed of the whole mess. For the first time since I had become pregnant, I didn't feel anxious about moving the wrong way or too fast. I felt as though a weight had been lifted.

The euphoria, the sense of regained control over my body and my life, lasted for exactly one week. During that week I convinced everyone I spoke with that I was FINE. After a few days of this, they all began to believe that I was back to normal, and they all returned to business as usual in their dealings with me. And then — without warning or precipitant — I crashed. I cried. I felt I couldn't stand it. I started feeling enraged that this had happened to me: I was angry that other people were going through their days normally while I was feeling the most intense grief I had ever known. A child of mine, along with all of the dreams, hopes, and fantasies I had for him, had died.

In the week following the miscarriage I began to mourn. The world lost its interest for me; I went through the motions of living feeling like a self-conscious, mechanical doll. I was aware of every move I made and every word I spoke, yet I didn't feel like me. I got up, I somehow struggled through the decision of what clothes to put on. I didn't bother with makeup because I had no energy to put it on, and it didn't matter what I looked like. I went downstairs and through the usual ritual of eating breakfast, but it didn't matter what went into my mouth; I hardly tasted the food. I would walk outside and drive to work daydreaming, in a daze. Much of the time I felt as though I were wrapped in a gauze dressing like a caterpillar in a cocoon. Nothing seemed to mean very much to me: I felt like an observer watching myself and everyone else going about the business of living, while I wandered around in a semi-invisible state. I was also pre-occupied with time. I counted the days over and over in an endless litany. How much time since the miscarriage; how long before we could start trying again; what fraction of the wait was over — down to the hour. Over and over and over and over.

The only thing that could draw me out of my deadness was when I could talk about what had happened to me. All of a sudden I became three-dimensional and animated, a complete person, alive. Of course the problem was that not everybody wanted to hear in full and vivid detail about every nuance of my miscarriage and its aftermath. In fact, very few people wanted to hear about it at all.

I began to feel a little crazy about needing to talk about it so much, and I think I may have used some unsuspecting people as listeners and sounding boards because I was so self-absorbed that I wasn't always aware of what the needs of the other person were. I was able to work fairly well, but during my nonworking hours I had a lot of trouble listening to other people's concerns. There were some people I couldn't speak to at all — most especially, pregnant friends. I could not stand to hear someone complain in any way, shape, or form about anything that had to do with being pregnant when I felt that if only I were pregnant, everything would be OK. Those friendships really suffered.

AUGUST 1979

Despite how horrible I felt during those months, I think few people noticed. I think that part of the intensity of the isolation I felt was that I could fool people so well. It was clear to me that most people wanted to believe that everything was fine. Everyone was only too willing to accept my superficial smile and work-as-usual schedule as evidence that things were back to normal.

I had never noticed before how there are a million things to remind one of pregnancy. A television commercial for Pampers would make me cry. A woman walking down the street in a loose dress would fill me with envy. As the days became longer and spring established itself, I could only think that I wasn't beginning to "show" the way I thought I would be when the buds and flowers started to bloom. I felt that every woman on the street could have something that I couldn't, something that I craved more intensely than I've ever desired anything in my life.

In addition, I was feeling exhausted. Everything seemed an incredible effort, from getting out of bed to washing my hair to dealing with my three-year-old son to picking up the telephone.

There was also less emotional energy than usual available for my child and my husband, because so much was consumed by my preoccupation with pregnancy. Although intellectually I knew that this was normal for someone as depressed as I, it nevertheless made me feel guilty.

My husband was as understanding as he could be, but he didn't comprehend what this had done to my whole sense of myself. He didn't understand why I wasn't consoled by the thought that I could have another pregnancy, and by already having one child. I worried about how little I had to give to our son. I felt at once overcome with our good fortune to have him and yet strangely angry with him and his demands.

It was a difficult time for my husband and me. I think that no matter how hard a woman tries to explain what it feels like to have her whole sense of herself as a creative being shaken, it is difficult if not impossible for a man to comprehend her experience on anything but an intellectual level. I'm sure that neither of us was prepared for how intensely upset I felt. After months of my moping and lack of interest, my husband finally confronted me with his feeling that by this time I should be able to have more perspective. I, of course, felt enraged by his insensitivity and resentful toward him for having escaped the full burden of the loss. I also felt confirmed in my sense of estrangement from him. In my heart of hearts, I began to wonder if the fault didn't lie with his sperm, rather than with my egg. Since that time I have learned that he suspected that the reverse was true. It seems that neither of us understood how deeply the loss had affected us individually and as a couple, and thus were unprepared for the many strong, and often irrational, feelings that emerged.

The very hardest single experience I had to face in the months after my miscarriage was a baby shower. The woman who invited me let me know sensitively that she would understand if I chose not to come, but that she wanted to give me the option of attending if I wanted to. Needless to say, it was a painful decision, and I was obsessed over what I should do until the hour at which I knew I'd have to leave if I were going to get there in time. I finally decided to go, in part because the guest of honor had herself been through a miscarriage, and she had talked endlessly with me about the depression and self-doubt that had followed for her, in part because it felt so self-indulgent and dramatic not to go that I knew it could only further lower my self-esteem if I gave in to the urge to bury myself for the duration. It was a sad evening for me. I had to try hard not to let my ever-present sadness show at such a joyous gathering. Yet how could there be anything else on my mind as I stared at my friend's ripe, round, beautiful body, and the proud bellies of several other of the guests as well. I felt shrunken, devalued, and useless, being unable to carry out this most wondrous of tasks.

I waited the required three months before putting away my diaphragm. Those first three periods were each welcomed with celebration, because it meant one less month to delay. Especially the first signaled to me that things were on their way back to normal, my body was cycling, and we hoped it would be a short time before we'd be trying to conceive again. Nevertheless, not being able to try when we wanted a baby so badly was extremely hard to tolerate. Time passed very slowly because I knew there was nothing to hope for.

We didn't conceive in the first cycle when we tried, and that was a big disappointment. It felt as though all the waiting and anticipation of the past four months built up to a climax in the days before my period was due. I even felt convinced that I was having symptoms of pregnancy. My mind played every trick: there was a little fullness to my breasts, a little nausea, a little extra tiredness. And then the blood came. I tried to pretend to myself that it wasn't really my period, that it was the kind of bleeding you can have and still be pregnant. When I could no longer pretend to myself that it wasn't really my period, I cried long and hard for the baby I had lost and the anguish I had felt, for the baby we hadn't started yet, and I cried for myself. It all came back in a giant, overwhelming rush — and I cried for it all, in frustration and helplessness, all over again.

POSTSCRIPT

JUNE 1980
It has been fifteen months since my miscarriage. Much of the writing was done during the time of my own bleak mourning, as an attempt to gain control of my feelings by putting them on paper, hoping to console myself as well as anyone who might someday read this. I am especially happy to be writing now that we have a second healthy son. I feel that I love him all the more for having gone through such hell before he came to us.

During the time I was pregnant with him, and particularly during the first trimester, I was unable to either look at or continue this account. In fact, I was almost too anxious to tell anyone that I was pregnant or to acknowledge to myself that this pregnancy felt totally different to me, and much more "right." I was quite sure that I could not bear to go through another miscarriage.

Now that it is behind me, I am happy to report that one does get over the anguish and the pain — if not completely, then enough to have the intensity of it dulled by the passage of time, and, it is to be hoped, by the birth of a child.

3

Stillbirth — The Death of a Child

Despite the best efforts of the medical profession, little is known about what causes stillbirth. More often than not, the pregnancy is normal and uneventful until, suddenly, fetal movement ceases, bleeding occurs, or labor starts.

The diagnosis is stillbirth, defined as the death of the fetus between the twentieth week of pregnancy and birth. Death may be detected while the fetus is still in the uterus, or possibly not until labor is underway, or until the baby is delivered. In the United States one stillbirth occurs for every eighty live births.

WARNING SIGNS

Women whose stillbirth is detected before labor begins frequently have a warning sign such as vaginal bleeding or cessation of fetal movement. They may experience pain in the pelvis, lower abdomen, or back. Or one or more of the symptoms of toxemia may be present: rapid, unexplained weight gain; swelling of the fingers, ankles, and eyelids; headache; or visual difficulties. At times, premature labor is the first danger signal.

If you are concerned that there might be a problem, you should call your doctor immediately. He or she will want to know as many details as possible, so that he or she can make an accurate assessment.

Reduced Frequency of Fetal Movement
Babies differ greatly in how active they are. However, if a particular baby becomes less active than it has been, this may be a warning

sign. Some doctors recommend charting fetal movements daily, over an hour period — for example, from six to seven o'clock each night — as a way of detecting early signs of fetal distress.

Bleeding
At any time during pregnancy, bleeding is a sign there may be trouble, yet the majority of women who bleed during pregnancy go on to carry the baby to term. If bleeding occurs, you should consult your doctor.

Pain
Persistent or severe pelvic pain such as cramping, heaviness, sharp stabbing, or contractions are other signs of trouble. Your doctor will want to know what type of pain you are having, how intense it is, and whether the pain is intermittent or constant.

Fetal Heartbeat
A significant sign of fetal life is a heartbeat, which can usually be detected with a fetoscope as early as the middle of the fifth month of pregnancy. As part of routine prenatal care, physicians listen for a fetal heartbeat. If the physician cannot find a heartbeat and suspects a stillbirth, he or she may order an ultrasound examination. This diagnostic aid allows him to visualize the fetus directly and to determine if a heartbeat is present. If a heartbeat still cannot be detected, stillbirth is then diagnosed.

COPING WITH THE FIRST SIGNS OF TROUBLE

Most women, when they see that first drop of blood, become concerned about pain, or realize that the baby has not moved for "too long," experience a "sinking feeling in the pit of the stomach." While they may fear that something is wrong, they may not want to face the possibility that they might lose the baby. It is common to feel emotionally frozen and to deny that there may be a problem — even to the extent of telling oneself that one was just imagining things. A woman probably considers phoning her doctor, but she may feel that she would be needlessly interrupting him, that she is being a "hysterical woman."

These are common reactions, but this is not the time for stoicism. She should tell her physician immediately if she is experiencing any of the warning signs. If the doctor cannot be reached, or is not responsive to the patient's concerns, it is wise to visit the emergency room of a good nearby hospital. It is better to err on the side of being too concerned.

The Bad News

If you have experienced symptoms and fear bad news, ask your husband or a friend or relative to accompany you to the doctor's office or the hospital. Your suspicions may be confirmed if the physician fails to detect a fetal heartbeat, or if he discovers that the uterus has failed to grow or has decreased in size, and if ultrasound examination fails to demonstrate the embryonic sac or the fetal heartbeat. If stillbirth is diagnosed, prepare yourself by asking your physician to describe what will happen, step by step. Your ability to cope with the physical and medical aspects of stillbirth will be improved if you are well informed. Your husband or a friend should hear this information as well, since it is possible that you may be feeling too upset to comprehend or remember very much.

SPONTANEOUS OR INDUCED LABOR

When stillbirth occurs prior to labor, the mother usually goes into labor spontaneously and delivers within about two weeks. However, this is not always the case. Sometimes labor may not begin for a month or more after stillbirth has occurred.

Because a woman who carries a dead fetus for more than four weeks has a 25 percent chance of developing a severe blood clotting disorder, known as intravascular coagulation, the pregnancy is always terminated well before the fourth week after intrauterine death.

Until recently, when stillbirth occurred prior to delivery, there was no alternative but to carry the pregnancy until labor began spontaneously, because there was no safe way to induce labor and cesarean section carried significant risks. Now, labor may be safely induced at any time after stillbirth is discovered using hormones called prostaglandins.

Carrying a stillborn baby until labor begins is an emotionally distressing experience that most women prefer to avoid. For this reason most women choose to have labor induced as soon as possible. However, such is not the case for everyone. Some women prefer to carry the pregnancy in the hope that labor will begin spontaneously before two or three weeks have passed. This alternative is chosen by some women who prefer that labor and delivery be as natural as possible, and by others who wish to be with their child as long as they can. The final choice should be left to the individual, unless there are overriding medical considerations.

In discussing her decision to have labor induced, Catherine said: "I previously had a miscarriage in which I spotted for three weeks before it ended. The waiting was terrible — they were days lost out of my life. Every day I lay on the couch and hoped and waited and sometimes cried. During my second pregnancy, when my doctor diagnosed stillbirth, I asked for labor to be induced as fast as possible, and I entered the hospital the next morning."

Another woman, Janet, chose to await spontaneous labor, explaining, "Rationally, I knew my baby had died (at eight and a half months), but I couldn't yet choose to start labor. My husband and I wanted time to get over the shock, if possible, before labor and delivery. As it turned out, we had six days before labor started. I cried and Roy and I comforted each other during those days. In the hospital, he stayed with me and helped me through labor and delivery, using the techniques we learned in a natural childbirth class. All along, we had wanted everything to be natural, and we stuck to that even though we knew the baby was dead."

LABOR AND DELIVERY

Because labor and delivery are events of great magnitude, you may have found yourself preoccupied by the physical aspects of what was happening to you. The considerable pain of labor and delivery may have absorbed you and led you to suppress your feelings about your baby's death until after delivery. On the other hand, you may have been constantly feeling emotional pain over your loss and the irony of going through labor and delivery. Many women are anxious about their lack of knowledge and preparation for labor and delivery, fear surgery in the case of a cesarean section, and are apprehensive about hospitalization.

Some women have felt that it was preferable to be awake and aware during the delivery of a stillbirth because it helped them to experience the reality of what happened. Others requested general anesthesia, though it is not medically feasible for everyone.

Women who have experienced warning symptoms or who have received the diagnosis of stillbirth before delivery are naturally better prepared for the bad news. Others who have enjoyed normal, uncomplicated pregnancies are stunned to find out during labor or delivery that the baby is dead. This is the most difficult time to learn about a baby's death. Their expectations were high then and they were happily anticipating seeing their baby soon. Learning of the baby's death at this time is a tremendous blow; when compounded by the pain of the birth, the combined impact may be overwhelming. In addition, the labor and delivery staff are in all likelihood unprepared for what happened, and therefore shocked, upset, and unable to offer the support the mother so badly needs.

VIEWING THE BABY

Shortly after delivery, parents may choose whether or not they wish to see their stillborn baby. Each couple must decide for themselves whether or not they choose to see or hold their dead infant. The most effective role of the staff is to avoid making the decision for the parents, but to support them in whatever decision they reach. Seeing the baby should not be imposed on them, but offered, as people have different feelings and these feelings should be respected.

Sarah and John decided to see their baby. Sarah described the experience: "My husband said it was a girl and she was really beautiful. He told me he thought I should see her and I said OK. I knew this was my only chance and I might be sorry later if I didn't. The nurse brought the baby in, all wrapped in a blanket. We both looked at her and touched her. She looked perfect, which was nice. It was a kind of a closure. We made a baby and she died."

Hospital practice and policy regarding seeing a baby that is dead varies tremendously. Many times the attitude of the individual doctor or nurse on duty determines how the situation is handled. Couples may either be encouraged to see the baby or discouraged from seeing it. In some instances, the matter is not brought up at all and must be initiated by the parents themselves. A couple has a right to see and hold their baby if they want to and should request to do so if the opportunity is not offered. Sometimes, if the baby has been dead for a few days, deterioration of the skin can occur; in other cases, the fetus may have a visible abnormality. Even in such instances, parents should be allowed to see the baby if they wish to. The staff should prepare them for what they will see. For many people, imagining the baby's appearance is very much worse than seeing and knowing.

One woman said: "Even though the baby was very tiny, I would have liked to have seen it at some point. I grieved so long for a baby with no face. I think seeing it would've helped me deal with the death better and I would've gotten over it faster. I used to stop and look at kids on the street and in stores and wonder if my child would've looked like that. People should have the option of seeing a dead baby. I would've liked to have seen it. I *still* would like to see it if I could."

For others, viewing the baby helps in the grief process. "It is much easier, I think, to grieve for a son, a person, seen, felt, touched, as opposed to not knowing. (And what a monstrous image we could have conjured up!) Seeing him erased my doubts of his existence or general condition. Seeing him helped to focus our grief — on someone who was."

Similarly, a young mother said: "I saw him. It was helpful. I wish I had a picture. He looked so peaceful, as if he was asleep, unlike the way I imagined him in his struggle with death."

However, some people choose not to view the baby and later feel it has been the right decision. Alice, a secretary, said: "We didn't want to see the baby. We felt it would be too hard on us, that it would imprint the death too strongly in our minds. My mother viewed the baby for us. She said she was beautiful and normal-looking. Somehow, her word was enough and a comfort to me."

In the last few years several hospitals have begun the practice of taking photographs of all stillborn babies. The photographs are given to the parents if they want them. If they do not, the pictures are kept, in case they wish to have them at some future time.

FUNERAL ARRANGEMENTS

Parents need to decide whether they want a religious ceremony, as well as how to deal with the stillborn baby's body. Many do not want the additional stress of having a ceremony and ask the hospital to take care of all the arrangements. For others, the process of making arrangements — deciding whether to have a ceremony, naming the baby, and deciding whether to have a headstone — is helpful. Some parents find that the gathering of supportive and sympathetic family members and friends at religious rites helps them deal with their grief. The ceremony may also underscore the reality of death and the finality of it, helping them to face their loss and to grieve.

Because the death of your stillborn may be the first death you have encountered in your family, you may be unaware of religious practices. Generally, Protestant and Catholic clergymen follow the desires of the parents regarding ceremonies for a stillborn baby, while the Jewish faith does not recognize a baby until after it is one month old, so no formal ceremony is available.

A funeral service for a stillborn child is rare. In some Protestant denominations, a memorial service is held, if desired, within several weeks or a month. Family and friends gather for prayers, hymns, and meditation, often centering on the joy of resurrection, in a spiritually uplifting service.

Some couples prefer only a simple graveside service where the body or ashes are interred.

A Catholic priest said he is sometimes called to the hospital following a stillbirth, where he prays with and comforts the parents. Most often, he is contacted by the husband or wife several weeks after delivery. "They will request a special mass to be attended by family and friends. It is part of their grieving process." Also possible is a graveside service. Here again, the emphasis is on what the parents want and need.

Some couples derive great comfort from a religious service. For others it is an ordeal to be suffered through. The decision to have a service or to avoid such things should be yours alone and your wishes should be respected.

THE HOSPITAL STAY

For those who have had a stillbirth, the hospital stay is often traumatic. You probably haven't forgotten one detail of your experience, and like many other women, you may wish you had done some things differently.

You may have been in the hospital for the first time in your life; doubtless you found hospital routines to be unfamiliar, upsetting, and intimidating. Possibly you preferred to do what you were told rather than to make your personal preferences known. Like most, you probably felt extremely vulnerable and had difficulty in arranging to have your needs met.

It is our experience that when women take control, their hospital stay tends to be a less painful one. Most people feel much less frightened if they know what to expect. It is always reasonable to request information about what has happened to you and about what is likely to happen next.

Most women find that having their husband, or a close friend or relative, with them during labor and delivery is helpful. It is routine practice in some hospitals to permit the husband to be with his wife during labor and delivery, or in the case of surgery, with her during premedication and recovery. In other hospitals, special permission may be required.

It is probably a good idea for *any* pregnant woman to consider whether, if the pregnancy should be lost, she would prefer to be separated from other obstetric patients during labor and recovery. If you would prefer your postpartum stay to be in the gynecology or surgical area, tell your doctor and hospital personnel and *insist* on getting what you want. Be prepared to be told that your request is "against hospital regulations" or that you are an "impossible patient." Ignore the temptation to back down and withdraw your request. Several days of seeing babies and happy parents can be far more unsettling than an irritated nurse or administrator.

Many women who recovered in the maternity ward found it extremely painful. "I was placed in a combination maternity-gynecology floor," said Karen. "This was a very emotionally upsetting experience. It might sound like I was trying to hide from the real world, but I found it very difficult to be surrounded by what

I couldn't have. It was almost as if someone was rubbing it in my face. I was on a happy floor and I was far from being happy. I learned very quickly to stay in my room with the door shut when the nursery cribs were being rolled past my door. In fact, I didn't like walking in the hall at all."

Seeing parents with their babies can be traumatic, some women feel. Sharing a ward with happy mothers caused some women to hide their feelings lest they spoil the happiness of others.

"I went home as soon as possible," one woman said. "There was a woman on the other side of the curtain with her family admiring their healthy baby. It tore me apart not to have mine."

Several women commented that they would have coped better if they had been in private rooms. "I wish I'd had a private room. I was unable to cry, so I held back my emotional feelings. I didn't want to disturb my roommate. I couldn't tell my husband how I felt, because my roommate was always there."

On the other hand, some women find that isolation in a private room adds to their feelings of failure, guilt, and misery. They are less lonely sharing a room with one or more women and think it is an advantage to be with others. "I was glad to have an understanding woman in the next bed. She was recovering from surgery. She listened to me and encouraged me to talk about how bad I felt. It was especially good to have her there late in the evening after my husband left."

Many couples who have experienced a stillbirth want to remain together throughout the hospital stay. If you want your husband to stay with you, you or he should negotiate this with the floor personnel. If you have a private room, the staff may be willing to put a cot in your room for him. In all likelihood there will be times when you feel you want to be by yourself or alone with your spouse; be sure to communicate this. Hospital personnel should respect your wish for privacy. Also, let them know whether you want visitors. If you want friends and relatives to have unrestricted visiting privileges, communicate this so it can be arranged.

It is reasonable to request that your doctor inform all hospital personnel on your floor about your situation so that you are dealt with appropriately. A thirty-year-old computer programmer related her experience after a stillbirth: "Nurses came in and asked me several times if I had a name for my baby yet. I couldn't believe they didn't read my chart to know what happened to me. I was still in shock and I couldn't believe I was in a maternity ward. I did OK in the hospital, but kind of mentally collapsed when I got home — the whole experience was a total nightmare."

The lack of communication with your doctor, nurses, and other hospital staff members can be troubling. "I feel that my medical needs were met; however, there was no support for my emotional needs," one young woman said. "The doctor and the hospital personnel seemed not to know what to say, so they just acted very 'professionally' towards me. If the staff had simply acknowledged the fact that I did feel emotional pain, or even at least acknowledged that I felt something, it could have helped."

The main criticism that couples who have experienced a fetal loss have about the care they received while in the hospital is that nursing and medical personnel were not sufficiently available to them. Feeling that the staff avoided them, rather than offering sympathy and emotional support, was common. Women report that one distressing aspect of hospitalization is the isolation they feel. The lack of attention to the tragedy that has befallen them is another. Repeatedly, women told us of the need to talk to someone, to have their feelings of intense sadness validated. Avoidance by the hospital staff exacerbated feelings of unworthiness and guilt.

"I had a terrible hospital experience," the mother of a stillborn baby said. "Few, if any, offered support. Some were not aware of the experience and no one talked about the death. I wanted to talk, but no one gave me the opportunity or freedom to."

Generally, couples were relieved and grateful when medical personnel responded with sympathy and concern. Many women praised the invaluable support that they received from their doctors and nurses. They were appreciative when staff members listened to them talk about their feelings or acknowledged that they had had a difficult experience. Most felt that when they were treated sympathetically and allowed to express their grief openly, they tended to feel better. As Donna said: "I was in a private room and felt isolated. Nurses and staff members came in to talk to me — to relate similar experiences. This helped me cope, knowing I wasn't alone.

"And my doctor talked to me several times in the hospital. He said that he realized what this pregnancy meant to us. Although he was reassuring about future pregnancy, he acknowledged the grief I felt for this one. He even said that this was a very sad time and that I should feel free to cry. For some reason, I needed his permission to cry and I will always be thankful for this man's understanding and kindness."

Sometimes medical personnel are reluctant to offer emotional support or to initiate discussion for fear of invading your privacy. It may be up to you to approach them.

THE POSTPARTUM PERIOD

The postpartum period is the time between delivery and the return of the pelvic structures to their nonpregnant state. Generally, this takes about six weeks. For women who have had normal pregnancies, it tends to be a time of adjustment. For women who have lost their babies, this period is exceptionally stressful, both physically and emotionally.

During her postpartum hospital stay of one to three days, a bereaved woman is often still in shock and only beginning to face the depth of her feelings of loss. In addition to the emotional distress that she feels at this time, she will probably also experience some physical discomfort. Physical discomfort may be hard for her to bear because her ability to cope with stress is impaired. In addition, it may be a reminder that her body has been preparing for motherhood and this preparation has been for nought.

Physical Concerns

LOCHIA The first physical process a woman is likely to experience is vaginal discharge (lochia) from the site of placental attachment to the uterus. This usually begins during delivery and continues for up to a month afterward. At first, the lochia will be red. Over a few weeks, it will change to brown and then to a yellow-white discharge.

AFTERPAINS Immediately after delivery the uterine muscles contract. This blocks exposed uterine blood vessels, keeping bleeding to a minimum. When this happens, many women will experience abdominal cramps much like menstrual cramps or labor pains. These cramps, or afterpains, are usually most intense right after delivery has occurred. Thereafter, they decrease in intensity and frequency. Some women have afterpains for a day or two following delivery.

EPISIOTOMY Like many women, you may find that the stitches and the healing incision from the episiotomy are so uncomfortable that you are unable to sit in a hard chair or on a car seat for three weeks or so. Sitting on a pillow or inflatable "doughnut" is helpful, as well as taking a warm tub or sitz bath in about four inches of water but without soap or bubble bath. Gently patting the perineal area with a soft, clean cloth may also help. It is preferable to take a shower, rather than a bath, during the first three weeks postpartum to avoid the possibility of infection.

MILK IN BREASTS Many women who have had a second-trimester miscarriage or a stillbirth find that on the second to fourth day after delivery their breasts become engorged with milk. Since one's body has no way of knowing that the fetus has died, it automatically prepares for breast feeding. Engorgement may cause some physical discomfort, but normally the actual physical pain is less troublesome than the emotional pain that may accompany it. Barbara described finding that her breasts were full of milk as "nature's cruel joke." Like many women, she was both surprised and horrified to find that her body was preparing to feed a child that would never be.

Sarah commented, "My breasts were bothering me, and when I would think of them being full of milk, sometimes tears would fill my eyes and sometimes I would feel angry. It seemed so unfair that I had all this milk, but no baby to feed it to. Something else that I found disturbing was that I had spent several months preparing my nipples and breasts for feeding, attended classes, expecting to nurse. Now in the hospital I was trying to stop the milk."

We would like to offer several suggestions for dealing with breast engorgement. First, you should not squeeze your breasts, since this will result in further production of milk. To relieve discomfort, wear a tight bra to bind the breasts, apply ice packs or hot wet compresses, or take an aspirin or other mild pain-relief tablet. The milk will soon dry up of its own accord.

Postpartum Blues

Most women are noticeably affected by the rapid and dramatic decrease in reproductive hormone levels which occurs at the time of delivery. Many experience physiological depression, irritability, and mood swings caused by hormone withdrawal; these feelings are commonly known as "milk blues." Usually the postpartum blues are relatively mild and short-lived; however, in a woman who has had a stillbirth, they can compound an already present grief reaction.

A happy mother with a healthy baby may suddenly find herself in tears because her emotional threshold is unusually low. However, chances are this is a time-limited problem and in a matter of days, or at most a few weeks, she will feel better. In contrast, the mother of a stillborn baby might find the combination of profound grief and physiological depression to be distressing and overwhelming. Weeks may pass with no decrease in the intensity of her emotions. She may feel depressed, out of control, irritable, and unable to cope.

Other Concerns

Generally, during the postpartum period women tend to feel fatigued and depressed. That is why it is important to get lots of rest. Seek help with whatever household or other tasks seem too much for you. And of course, you should recuperate fully before returning to your job and a demanding schedule.

Sexual relations can be resumed three weeks after delivery if the stitches have healed, the vagina is not painful, and all bleeding and discharge have stopped.

Normally, your first menstrual period will start in about a month to two months after delivery.

Any unusual signs or symptoms should be reported to your doctor. These include fever, with or without chills; heavy vaginal bleeding; unusual breast or abdominal pain; and painful urination.

LOSING WEIGHT Following stillbirth a number of women report difficulty coping with the weight gain of pregnancy and with still "looking pregnant," because the increased weight and change in body contours were associated with the baby inside them. Some women become obsessed with losing weight and getting back to their nor-

mal size. They join exercise classes and go on strict diets in an effort
to erase at least the physical signs of the failed pregnancy. They may
gain some satisfaction in the ability to control this one facet of their
lives, feeling that everything else is out of their hands. Other women
may lack interest in their weight and appearance. Because they feel
depressed, they may use food as a source of satisfaction. Whatever
your reaction, your diet and exercise plan should be checked out
with your doctor and any rapid loss or gain of weight avoided.

CAUSES OF STILLBIRTH

Once a stillborn baby is delivered, parents and medical staff members try to determine what caused the death. Among the known
causes of stillbirth are chromosomal abnormalities, umbilical cord
accidents, placental problems, and toxemia. However, it is not uncommon that no cause is found, even after an examination of fetal
and placental tissues and an autopsy of the infant.
   Stillbirth occurs at the rate of 10.4 for every 1,000 live births.
   The following chart shows the presumed cause of stillbirth.

Fetal anoxia	21%
Congenital malformations	8%
Unknown causes	32%
Maternal pathological conditions	20%
Inappropriate fetal growth	13%
Systemic fetal infection	6%

(Statistics taken from Y. W. Brans, M. B. Escobedo, et al., "Perinatal Mortality in a
Large Perinatal Center: Five-year Review of 31,000 Births," *Am. J. Obstet. Gynecol.* 148,
No. 3 [1984]: 284–289.)

Cord Accidents
Umbilical cord accidents pose a threat to a fetus because they may
cause the oxygen supply through the cord to be cut off. Sometimes
the cord develops a knot or coils around the fetus's neck or body so
tightly that oxygen is shut off or interrupted, resulting in either
fetal death or damage. Most cord accidents occur during labor and
delivery, although they can cause intrauterine death prior to labor.
They are unlikely to happen to the same mother more than once.

Placental Disorders

Severe placental problems can cause fetal death. In placenta previa, the placenta is implanted low in the uterus instead of in its normal location high on the anterior or posterior (front or back) wall of the uterus. Evidence of placenta previa is usually painless vaginal bleeding in the last trimester of pregnancy. The blood is bright red and the flow may range from light to heavy. The baby is unaffected unless the mother's blood loss is severe and results in a decrease in the oxygen supply to the fetus.

Another placental problem is premature separation of the placenta from its site of implantation in the uterus. Separation is considered premature if it occurs anytime before delivery. It is most common in the third trimester, but can happen at any time after twenty weeks. The seriousness depends on whether the separation is partial or complete. Placental separations range from very partial ones, which may be largely asymptomatic and have no evident effect on the fetus, to severe separations, which lead to excruciating uterine pain, hemorrhage, and fetal death.

Genetic Factors

Genetic studies should be carried out to determine whether either parent or the fetus carries a chromosomal abnormality. If this is the case, genetic counseling is advised before another pregnancy is conceived.

Preeclampsia and Eclampsia (Toxemia)

Severe toxemia is a major cause of perinatal death and can lead to maternal death as well. There is no known cause of toxemia. Symptoms may include sudden and excessive weight gain; swelling of the fingers and ankles; puffiness of the eyelids; headache; and disturbances in vision. The majority of women with early preeclampsia, however, are not symptomatic. Because elevated blood pressure and protein in the urine can usually be detected before any overt symptoms are present, it is important that all women have frequent obstetric visits late in gestation. When it is diagnosed in its early stages and medical advice is followed, the more severe consequences of this disorder can be prevented.

Other Factors
There are many other factors that may cause stillbirth, including maternal illness, either infectious or systemic (such as diabetes); complications of labor or delivery; Rh factor incompatibility (almost always preventable), and severe nutritional deficiency.

One Woman's Story

One year later. Somehow it seems like only yesterday. The weather is much the same — naturally — though it is hard to recall much about the weather then. Only that during my labor (in August) I somehow convinced the nurse to turn on the heat and bring blankets. And the way it rained, soft and cool and so green, the day they buried the baby.

I had a very easy pregnancy — only the most minor complications — had no morning sickness — felt and looked remarkably healthy. Starting from the first visit to the doctor, at ten weeks, there was not the slightest hint of any difficulty. My chart consistently showed "o" risk. There were of course the jokes and rebukes about my weight gain, which was considerable. Not to say those visits were easy — the doctors always seemed concerned and helpful — but there was always the nagging thought "Does he remember me, or know my name without referring to my chart?" Perhaps it was sheer unreasoned anxiety, simply a case of being overwhelmed by one's emotions. Later, my hand would shake at the prospect of telephoning his office.

On the last scheduled doctor's visit before my due date I was full of eager anticipation. The nursery was set and I was looking forward to taking my leave from the office and having a few days at home for final preparations. (I fully expected to deliver late). It was a summer day like many others. As was our usual routine, it was a late morning appointment, to be followed by lunch with my grandparents. Joseph dropped me off and left to do his usual errands.

My doctor's partner was on duty, and I went into his examining room, where the baby's heartbeat would be broadcast on a speaker near the table. Like always. First, the casual greetings. I told the doctor I hadn't noticed the

*baby moving for a couple of weeks. The doctor explained this was not un-
common at this stage, due to the larger size of the baby. He checked last
Saturday's report — oh yes, Dr. B. had found movement.*

*Then the stethoscope was ready . . . no familiar sound . . . the phone rang,
and the doctor casually left to reassure some other expectant mother. Soon he
was back, and patiently resumed the search for the elusive heartbeat. Then he
stopped.*

*I was confused, and asked naively, "Is this cause for concern?" He as-
sured me it was. He manipulated my belly but got no response. He would not
say anything; he only scheduled another appointment and remarked that he
hoped I wouldn't still be waiting then.*

*Tears filled my eyes as I spoke with the nurse on the way out. I was
confused, fearful, but not sure. Was the baby dead? If so, why hadn't the
doctor told me?*

*Joseph was waiting, and I got into the car. In his usual fashion he would
have had us at my grandparents' door in a half-minute, but I begged him to
detour and find a place where we could sit and talk. I needed time to compose
myself and tell him. We were still not sure. But we agreed not to tell my
grandparents. Once there, we said little, and I went to the bathroom to cry
as often as I could, and put on my best effort so as not to alarm them.*

*We left as soon as we could. I told Joseph there are times when only one's
mother will do. We went to my parents' house, and Joseph told my father as
I cried in the bathroom. My mother was at the town common at one of the
local festivities, Autumn Fair.*

*We set out to find her. Searching through the crowd, my eyes found her in
a lawn chair in a shady spot. I explained what had happened, and she, too,
was concerned. A neighbor whose wife was due about the same time came by
with a bright smile and cheery remarks. She shooed him away. We hugged for
a while, and when I felt strengthened, Joseph took me home.*

*It was then I decided that one point of our childbirth classes had been the
helpfulness of the nurses. Rather than endure this uncertainty, I called the
labor and delivery unit. By luck Mrs. L., the head nurse, answered. I didn't
know her then, only that there was a calm, understanding, patient woman at
the other end of the line. I explained what had happened at the doctor's office,
and asked her opinion. She erased my uncertainty and let me down very
gently.*

*"Why didn't the doctor tell me?" I asked. "You know, we're human,
too. . . ." She wondered why the doctor hadn't informed her. Quick to defend*

him, I explained that it had only been a few hours since my appointment. Anyway, she asked a few questions and reassured me that she would be expecting me. I didn't quite grasp the importance of that until later.

So I began to get used to the idea. Try as I might, I could no longer stimulate any movement from within. At last there was no hope, and I had to think of what to do, to plan.

Mother called. She had discussed my case with a nurse friend, and had gotten an answer of little hope, but maybe a slight chance. She, like me, was grasping at straws. Now it was my turn to gently explain how I had talked to the nurse in labor and delivery, and that I no longer doubted. She didn't give up, though. She had talked to both my doctor and his partner at length by noon the next day, pressing them for answers.

Somehow the rest of the day and evening passed. I was determined to stay in the house — no more public places and friendly faces and cheery remarks. They meant well, of course, but I couldn't bring myself to risk the confrontation.

Joseph was very good. He came to understand even more slowly than I, and somehow buried his personal torment in his concern for me. He was anxious to throw himself into some sort of activity, but he refused to leave me alone.

Sunday midday. I sat on the deck soaking up the sun and trying not to think.

By Sunday afternoon Joseph arranged to take me to my mother's house for a while, and he then got away for a little. I sat in a nice straight-back chair and faced the television. We didn't talk much. It had gotten down to waiting. . . .

Back home, after dinner, there were at last decisions to be made. I had planned to work this week. My due date was Friday, but I had felt good, and had wanted to have the time off after the baby came rather than before. Moreover, I expected to be late. So my car pool was expecting me. On Saturday the doctor had said I could still go to work, but now the thought was appalling. So I decided that now was the time to get ready: wash hair, shave, and be ready. This done, my efforts at procrastination were about exhausted, and by nine o'clock I finally called a fellow in the car pool. I sadly explained that I would not be in, and would call when ready to return, sooner than I had planned.

We went to bed around ten. Now I was really hoping the time would come soon, that I would be spared this horrible waiting much longer. The lifeless *baby was by now a burden, a source of frustration, such as he had never been in nine months. In the past I had chided him gently if he kicked a lot — now I would have given anything to feel such a little discomfort. Now he was just a lump, like a sack of potatoes. I hoped my time would come soon.*

Mercifully we slept soundly until I was awakened by a sharp pain at 12:45 A.M. I was greatly relieved and was sure this was it. Before I had wondered if I would recognize the onset of labor. I had felt the Braxton Hicks contractions a lot late in my pregnancy, and once thought that might be what labor was. The doctor had laughed at my concern — after all, every woman knows. It feels like a contraction — well, how was I to know what a contraction feels like? It was not like anything I had experienced in the past, but I didn't press him too much because, after all, he never felt one, either. My sister had described hers, and her description was concrete enough, and exactly fit what I felt now. The bloody "show" was simply confirmation of what I already knew.

I called Mother and arranged for her to call our offices in the morning. Joseph was very nervous, and tried to rush me. But I lingered, fretting over the contents of my suitcase, sadly lacking baby things, only what I needed, and didn't need, for myself. I was terribly thirsty. Joseph made glass after glass of iced tea. Finally I was ready, and we set out for the hospital. At that point the pains were sharp but very short, and came at irregular but short intervals.

It didn't take long to get to the hospital. It was very dark and the roads were empty. We went to the emergency entrance as instructed. A nice little old man put me in a wheelchair, and, unknowing, tried to console me as I cried all the way to the maternity ward. Joseph followed after he had taken care of some paperwork.

The nurse was very nice and tried to cheer me up. "You're going to have a baby!" As I undressed in a little bathroom, Joseph quietly told her the unhappy circumstances. She then calmly prepped me, and in a perfunctory way put the stethoscope on my belly — no sound — for just the shortest time. Then I wanted to get up and move around. She sent us both in our white gowns to the fathers' waiting room. This room faced the nursery. We looked through and paced the floor and talked with a father-to-be who asked about my progress and told how his wife was doing. We didn't tell him.

Soon, the nurse came back and escorted us away from that depressing situation. We had asked for a private room, and she took us there now. It was a lovely large room, with one semicircular wall, all windows, overlooking a grassy area with trees. I remember especially the flowered wallpaper, which I would try to use later as a focal point for concentration.

I got into bed, with ginger ale and lollipops close by. Joseph settled into a comfortable chair, and we dozed. When the pains came, I called him to my side, and he always came, to help me, and when they subsided we napped again. Over and over from about 2 A.M. to daylight.

I remember the strangeness of the pains. When I got a strong one, I can remember thinking, This is the most horrible feeling in the world, and wondered how many children would be born if men had to bear them. At the same time, as the pain subsided, the relief was great. And when the pain was gone, it was just about forgotten. Was it really so bad?

Several times I had to go to the bathroom. Joseph's voice outside the door, over and over, queried, "Are you all right?" It was reassuring.

By morning the pains were getting stronger and Joseph valiantly tried to time them. I paid little attention, but often asked, "How often is it now?" At seven the doctor on duty was the same who on Saturday had found no life inside me. He advanced no farther than the doorway. Mrs. L., who had checked me shortly before, came with him. He asked two questions. He asked about the progress of my labor, to which Mrs. L. answered something, and he asked me if "anything had changed." I said only "no" and felt miserable. The look on his face, as Joseph later described it, was the look of death, an expression we shall never forget. I expect he felt truly sad — but at the time I was kind of disappointed that he didn't show more concern for me, that he did not examine me or even step towards me in the room.

In another way I was a little glad to think that this was his final round, and that my regular doctor would be on duty when I delivered.

Mrs. L. came in again. My mother had called, and she spoke with her. Again I felt reassured, not alone.

On one visit, Mrs. L. took over Joseph's job and helped me through a contraction. I was amazed at how much help another person could be. The other nurses had been nice, but lacked her authority. Even Joseph, whom I never promised to "obey," was less effective in this role. The adaptation of deep breathing — she taught me to let my belly rise on the inhale, hold, and fall on exhale — was much better for me than anything we did in childbirth class. Or maybe it was just her.

By eight o'clock I told Joseph I was losing my concentration and to ring for the nurse. Mrs. L. had just left, but the contractions were much stronger. Now she stayed with me. Into heavy labor. She checked me, positioned me, and leaned over me very close as we breathed together. It was as if we were one person. Soon it was really happening. I told her, "I feel something coming," and she said, "Let it go." It was the bag of waters breaking. She competently cleaned up. Now I really couldn't control — just let my head back in a kind of loud noise, more like a great groan than a scream. She pushed my head back down. "Don't let it out — push." It was at that time, about 8:30, she got the table and we went down to the delivery room. She advised Joseph to stay behind since she didn't expect it to be much longer. I was going to be given gas, as we had requested.

But I fooled her. I was not so eager as other women, knowing the outcome. We were in the delivery room for an hour before they finally put me under.

For some reason I thought the anesthetist and the doctor would not arrive in time. Anyway, I was not doing my best to hurry things along. I tried to sleep. I tried breathing instead of pushing. Watching the clock on the wall, I hoped it would be over soon, that I would be asleep and unaware of the rest.

Mrs. L. kept working on me. She called the doctor and the anesthetist. After a while I could see my doctor outside the delivery room. I could see his capped head over the top of a partition in front of the door. So he would not be late after all.

Finally at about 9:30 they all converged on me and decided I was ready. I felt like so much hamburger lying on the table, but felt relieved that the time had come and that these people would take care of me. I was just starting to fade out when I could feel a cool mist sprayed on my bottom — just a little bit of panic — I moved to show them I was still conscious, and someone said, "Wait a minute" — then I remember no more.

Awake and shaking, I saw only Mrs. L. still in the room. She was over near the wall in front of me doing something at a table. Joseph came in. He let out a scream, reeled, and punched the wall. She had shown him the baby. She ordered me to keep my head down.

Earlier Mrs. L. had asked if we wanted to see the baby. We had said no, but she advised us it would be better. Now I realized how right she was.

Joseph moved over by me, tears still in his eyes, and Mrs. L. gently brought the baby to me to hold. Like any other couple, our first question was "What is it?" A boy. And then, "How big?" Six pounds.

He had only been dead two or three days, so he looked very good — beautiful, as if asleep — wrapped in a blanket. Mrs. L. said not to open the blanket, as some skin had begun to deteriorate, but that there was no apparent abnormality. I held him for several minutes. I saw that he had Joseph's

*dark hair, and a little bow mouth. I felt stunned. I didn't know what to say
or do. There were no tears then, just a sort of confused exhaustion, of being
overwhelmed by this sad event.*

*I know now what I should have done — I sorely regret not having kissed
him. Such a little thing. It just didn't occur to me until later, when it was too
late. We also should have given him a name. He was and is very real to
us — our son — but we had not agreed on a name before, and once we
learned his sad fate, we somehow couldn't bring ourselves back to the question of a name. He should have had a name. We will forever now refer to
him as "the baby." "The baby's room" is the nursery, his room, though he
never slept in it.*

*Basically, we were ill prepared to cope with death. We both had been
sheltered from other deaths, and had not suffered the loss of anyone close. So
this was by far the greatest loss of our lives, not even close to any other.*

*I lay there gazing at the baby and finally Mrs. L. took him away and
prepared me to return to my room. I was sort of relieved (I admit with some
guilt) because it was just so sad, and I felt so powerless, so frustrated and
confused.*

*We went back to my room about 11 o'clock and soon a nurse brought me
lunch. I was hungry in spite of everything and ate most of it. Right away they
wanted to know the name of the undertaker. This was another thing we had
blocked from our minds and so were now shaken and had no answer. I got
Joseph to call my mother for the name of the family friend, so that was taken
care of. Joseph called his parents. We had decided not to tell them until after,
since they live far away and there seemed no point in upsetting them any
earlier. I had told my parents and my sister, and my mother told my grandparents and the people at our offices.*

*That afternoon I slept. Joseph roamed the hospital and went home to
change. I ate my supper, and then worried that Joseph hadn't eaten. My
mother came to visit, and my sister and her husband, whom I asked to take
Joseph down to the cafeteria. Somehow concern over other things relieved a
little of the greater grief. We both responded to the visitors — it gave us a
chance for conversation, made us feel loved, and generally kept us going.*

*Joseph was allowed to stay past regular visiting hours, until about 10,
when I went to bed.*

*Tuesday morning early I was awakened by the sound of babies crying. I
wondered if any of the mothers were telling their babies not to cry, I thought
how wonderful it would have been if my baby could cry.*

My doctor came by around 7 and we talked. He said there was no apparent cause of the baby's death. He said I was fine and could go home soon — not today, as I suggested, but preferably tomorrow morning. I accepted his advice.

I specifically asked him whether he thought Rh incompatibility had been a problem. I knew that my blood type was B negative, that the Red Cross had told me I also had an antibody, anti-D, but that the blood test at twelve weeks had not shown the antibody. Joseph's blood type is B positive.

I had no other blood tests until after delivery. At delivery I was not given RhoGAM [a preparation of immune globulin which prevents the production of anti-Rh-positive antibodies in the mother's blood]; the doctor said now that I was already sensitized [if antibodies are already present RhoGAM is ineffective]. The doctor said that blood disease was not the cause of the baby's death, that had that been the case there would be evidence, but that may be a problem in future pregnancies. An autopsy would be done, but the doctor was not hopeful of finding an answer — "Many times they don't."

The issue of blood type incompatibility would continue to haunt us, probably because that was the only questionable item of my health. I had brought the Red Cross letter on my first visit to the doctor, and at that time he ordered the hospital test, and said I would be retested later near term. The hospital's test did not show the antibody, and when I asked the doctor about it he said one of the two was wrong, probably the Red Cross. When it got to be close to my due date, I had asked each of the doctors if I would be retested. Each said no. It appeared to us that they were relying solely on the hospital's test, which was proven wrong in the end. Now we were told it was not the cause of death, but still it is a source of nagging doubt, and a problem for the future as well.

Joseph spent most of Tuesday with me, except for the visit to the cemetery he arranged, with the undertaker and our friend Bob. They went to see different sites, to decide on one, and to order a monument. He decided on a family plot where my great-grandparents are buried. There was room enough, the location is a quiet corner, and it seemed nicer not to bury the baby alone. The stone was to have a cross, Baby Boy A., and the date. We felt that in two or three weeks, by the time the stone was laid, we would be ready to go there for a brief service. My sister's husband is a minister and we asked him to lead the prayers.

One of my friends called. From the fellows in my car pool, the news had worked its way around to my former work location. I asked her to come visit and she did that evening. My parents both came, so for another day we were glad to have visitors, and loads of flowers and cards. Some I got later at home, and they were very important to us. We got all kinds of cards — sympathy, get well, cheer up — and personal notes. The words hardly mattered. It was the idea that these people cared and took the time to try to express their sadness and concern for us. I have saved them to this day.

Joseph left late again Tuesday night. That was the only complaint of my hospital stay — that he had to go at all. I missed him each night and wished that he could have slept there with me. And he was unhappy going home alone.

The nurses were very good to us. Each was friendly and helpful on their periodic visits. Mrs. L. was my special nurse, and with about thirty years' experience and six children of her own, she really knew the situation. Besides taking me through my labor and giving us the baby, she also made my bed and watched me closely. She hugged me and cried with me. It was like being under total care — physical and mental. I left her some of my flowers and later sent some fruit as a token, albeit inadequate, of our appreciation for her extraordinary care. Come to think of it, she watched us both — as she wheeled me to the delivery room, she ordered another nurse to get Joseph a glass of orange juice with sugar, because he looked pale.

Wednesday morning. I awoke early to the sound of babies crying. Today was the day I could go home. It was also the day the baby would be buried. I looked out at the rain and the green grass and cried.

The doctor came by as I finished my breakfast. There was no further information, just instructions on postpartum care. The printed instructions were for women in happier circumstances, of course. One part begun, "When the baby is ten days old . . ."

I called Joseph and asked him to hurry. Finally he arrived and we prepared to leave. I had been dreading this moment. It seemed so sad to walk out empty-handed, past the glass-walled nursery. I clutched Joseph's arm and whimpered softly all the way to the car.

Home again. My sister and her husband came to see us that afternoon. Visitors again helping us by.

Wednesday night my milk came in. Tossing around in bed, there was this wetness. It seemed such a cruel blow that Mother Nature should do this to me now. Fortunately it didn't last, since I had had a shot in the hospital and had followed the nurse's advice.

Joseph stayed home with me and didn't go back to work until the following Monday. We had some visitors; mostly we stayed home. I felt safe being home.

I dreaded going out, fearing I would see someone I knew, or that anyone might ask about the baby. I still looked pregnant — and I still walked like a pregnant woman. My reflection in a storefront window was enough to reduce me to tears.

When Joseph went back to work I found that for the first time I was alone for significant periods. I began to really learn the meaning of words — like anguish. *In my mind's eye I saw Edward Munch's painting titled, I think,* The Scream. *That describes it better than words, and I felt it. I was more vulnerable now, since Joseph had hidden from me such things as the invoice for the baby's monument. Now I opened the mail alone — to find the bill from the undertaker, to find more cards, to find the final bill for the baby's monument. While all of this was hard to bear — I would cry, tear my hair — it was also a kind of catharsis that I was only able to accomplish when alone. I have a tendency to try to spare others my grief — if anyone asked about me, I would always answer "fine" or at least "OK." Chin up, good front, and all that. Some maybe felt I suffered less because it didn't show too much. In any case it is true that I felt almost apologetic if a friend started to cry or evidenced sadness on my behalf. So it was really in this time alone that I had to face what had happened, and overcome the great desire to hide forever.*

I would have six weeks' total leave, so by the end of two weeks I started to go daily to a health spa. Also on Fridays I went into town to lunch with my working friends (I would arrange to meet them at the restaurant, so as to avoid seeing any other people I knew). Once a week or so I lunched with my mother, who would pick up some sandwiches on the way. The days fairly flew by as I occupied considerable time on these simple activities.

A few times I was aware how little people understand about these things. One friend (mother of two) at lunch remarked how with all this spare time I must be getting all my fall cleaning done. I simply said no. Couldn't she see it was the farthest thing from my mind? The minister surprised me, too. He stopped in to see me at the hospital. He prayed for me and Joseph and we talked. I had to ask him point-blank to say a prayer for the baby. While I appreciated his concern for us, it is, after all, the baby's death we are mourning.

My faithful visits to the figure salon had little effect, although I did try. I was to learn much later that the weight loss I sought would come chiefly with time (one year) and little or no effort. Another of life's mysteries.

The Sunday three weeks from the baby's birth the stone had been set and we had our memorial service. My grandparents, parents, brother, sister, and our friend Bob (who was to have been the baby's godfather) came, and my sister's husband led us in prayer. I brought an arrangement of white flowers. It was simple and personal and I cried straight through. It was the first time I had been to the gravesite, though I have been often since.

One year later, we went again, Joseph and I, and placed yet another all-white arrangement at the baby's grave. And marveled at how it doesn't seem like a year has passed.

4 🎏

Ectopic Pregnancy —
A Compound Loss

"I had no warning. In fact, I had no idea what was going on until the emergency room nurse said it was an ectopic — a pregnancy in my right fallopian tube. Only then did it fit together. It was amazing how the shocky state I was in made me actually feel good and the deeper in shock I went, the better I felt.

"I realized at that point that there was nothing I could do to help myself or my husband. I knew he was very worried. It wasn't until several days after the surgery, when I was told that my chances of another ectopic were one in ten, that I began to comprehend what had happened to me and to feel the loss. Knowing I only had one tube left hit me very hard. I felt like my body had failed me.

"I felt frustrated and defeated. My husband was very distraught. He, more than I, realized how close to death I was. He was not willing to risk my life again for that of a possible baby."

Ectopic pregnancy. Before you had one you probably never heard of it. While you were in the middle of it you were probably stunned. You may have recently found out or not even have known you were pregnant. Then, suddenly, you were being rushed into the operating room. You woke up and learned that you had lost a baby and a fallopian tube. That's a tremendous loss, especially all at once. You are bewildered. "Why me?" you ask. "It's just not fair."

In the aftermath, you discovered very little is commonly known about ectopic pregnancy; many people you tell about it have never heard of it.

WHAT IS AN ECTOPIC PREGNANCY?

An ectopic pregnancy occurs when the fertilized egg implants itself outside the uterine cavity. By far the most common ectopic location is the fallopian tube (oviduct). This occurs in 95 percent of cases. Less commonly, the fertilized egg may implant in the ovary, the abdomen, or the cervix. Because it is most common, we will deal primarily with tubal pregnancy. Tubal pregnancy occurs approximately once in every 100 pregnancies in the United States.

Fertilization of the egg by the sperm usually occurs in the outer third of the fallopian tube. In a normal pregnancy, the egg is moved along through the tube by wavelike contractions and by the motion of hairlike cells, called cilia, which line the tube. After a journey of about two and one-half days, the egg reaches the uterine cavity, where it implants itself. If the passage of the egg through the tube is obstructed in any way, it is possible that the fertilized egg may implant in the tube instead of proceeding on to the uterus.

If the egg implants in the tube, it may establish a placenta and begin to grow just as if it were in the uterus. This initial growth of the embryo can trigger the placenta to produce the hormones of pregnancy. If this happens, the usual signs of pregnancy may be present: missed menstrual period, breast fullness and tenderness, and nausea. The hormones produced by the ectopically implanted placenta may also induce uterine growth and softening of the cervix, so that a physician may be unable to distinguish it from a normal uterine pregnancy.

As the embryo grows, the tube expands initially; however, since it is not capable of marked expansion, continued growth will cause it to rupture. The extent to which the pregnancy develops and the way it terminates depends, in part, on where in the tube the implantation has occurred. Tubal pregnancies terminate in a variety of ways. If the fertilized egg dies in the tube prior to implantation, or if it dies soon after implantation has occurred, the embryo may be reabsorbed (through the blood vessels) without damaging the tube or causing any symptoms. If the embryo dies but is not reabsorbed, mild chronic symptoms, most characteristically anemia, may occur. If ectopic pregnancy is diagnosed before the tube ruptures, the embryo can be surgically removed, saving the tube. Tubal rupture occurs when the growing embryo breaks through the tubal wall, or when the trophoblast, the primitive placenta, invades and erodes the blood vessels of the tube, causing hemorrhage. This usually occurs about two weeks after the missed menstrual period or four weeks after conception. Rupture of the fallopian tube is a medical emergency and requires immediate surgery.

RUPTURED TUBAL PREGNANCY — SIGNS AND SYMPTOMS

Diagnosis of an unruptured ectopic pregnancy is extremely difficult because the majority of patients do not develop clearcut signs and symptoms. When a pregnant woman develops severe abdominal pain in the first trimester, the possibility of ectopic pregnancy is usually considered. However, this possibility is sometimes overlooked when a woman who does not know she is pregnant experiences severe abdominal pain. If ectopic pregnancy is suspected, a very sensitive pregnancy blood test (measuring the beta subunit of HCG — human chorionic gonadotropin) is done. This test can detect the low level of hormones produced by the ectopic pregnancy. If the beta subunit test is positive, a sonogram (a picture made with ultrasound) will be done to see if the fetal sac is located in the uterus.

Most of the signs and symptoms of tubal pregnancy are caused by stretching, the ultimate rupture of the tubal wall, and hemorrhage into the tube or into the abdomen.

Pain
This is the most common symptom of a ruptured tubal pregnancy. Pain may be localized on one side or present over the entire abdomen. It may be cramping, stabbing, or tearing, intermittent or continuous. Commonly, the pain extends upward to the shoulder or neck. It may be the first symptom noted, or it may occur along with or after bleeding.

Missed Menstrual Period
Seventy-five percent of women with ectopic pregnancies report missing a menstrual period. One quarter of the patients report that

they did not miss a menstrual period. The bleeding associated with a tubal pregnancy may be mistaken for a normal period.

Vaginal Spotting and Bleeding
Vaginal bleeding is usually scanty and dark brown, and it may be intermittent or continuous. Severe vaginal bleeding rarely occurs in ectopic pregnancies. Profuse vaginal bleeding is more characteristic of miscarriage than of ectopic pregnancy, yet it occurs in 5 percent of all such cases.

Fainting and Weakness
These symptoms occur in about one third of women with ruptured tubal pregnancies and are caused by severe pain and hemorrhage.

Pain during Intercourse
Pain during intercourse sometimes is experienced with an ectopic pregnancy. Pain may result when the distended tube is jarred or when internal bleeding has occurred.

WHAT AN EXAM SHOWS

During a pelvic examination, movement of the cervix may cause severe pain. In 50 percent of patients, a tender pelvic mass can be identified to the side of or behind the uterus.

If bleeding has been significant, either into the abdomen or vagina, a decrease in blood pressure, an increase in pulse rate, and a drop in body temperature may result.

DIAGNOSIS

Because of the danger of hemorrhage, it is important to know the warning signs and to report them promptly when they occur. Since the consequences of a ruptured ectopic pregnancy are serious, it is best to err on the side of safety and to check out all concerns with your obstetrician.

Some other conditions mimic some of the signs and symptoms of ecoptic pregnancy: pelvic inflammatory disease, threatened or incomplete miscarriage, an ovarian cyst, and appendicitis. The physician will take a detailed history, perform a physical examination, and probably also order some tests to help him make a diagnosis. Following are some of the tests used.

Common Diagnostic Procedures

CULDOCENTESIS Insertion of a needle through the vagina into the space behind the uterus to determine whether there is blood in the abdominal cavity. The presence of blood would indicate that tubal rupture has occurred.

POSTERIOR COLPOTOMY A surgical incision made in the vaginal wall to investigate whether blood has accumulated in the space behind the uterus. If it has, this is a sign that the tube has ruptured and that internal bleeding has occurred.

CULDOSCOPY Visualization of the abdominal cavity by means of an instrument inserted through an incision in the vagina.

LAPAROSCOPY A procedure in which an optical instrument called a laparoscope is inserted through a small incision in the abdominal wall. This procedure permits the doctor to visualize directly the fallopian tubes and other pelvic organs.

ULTRASONOGRAPHY Use of high-frequency, short-wavelength sound-wave reflections to determine whether the uterus is enlarged, whether a fetus can be visualized in the uterus, and whether an ectopic fetal mass can be distinguished outside the uterus.

PREGNANCY TEST In recent years pregnancy tests have become of greater value in diagnosing ectopic pregnancies. With early gestation only small amounts of the pregnancy hormones are produced, so it is not uncommon for a woman with an ectopic pregnancy to have a negative routine pregnancy test. Recently, however, the test for the beta subunit of HCG, described previously, has been available to aid in the diagnosis of ectopic pregnancy. Because it is able to measure lower levels of pregnancy hormones than could be determined by ordinary pregnancy tests, an ectopic pregnancy can usually be ruled out if this test is negative.

Treatment

Surgery is required whenever ectopic pregnancy is diagnosed or strongly suspected, even if the tube has not ruptured. Salpingectomy (removal of the entire fallopian tube) is the surgical procedure most frequently performed. Conservative surgery — that is, an effort to repair or reconstruct the damaged tube — is performed when the woman wishes to attempt pregnancy in the future and her other tube is nonfunctioning or absent, while the damaged tube appears to be salvageable.

There is, unfortunately, an increased risk of having a recurrent ectopic pregnancy after conservative surgery because adhesions or scar tissue may form and obstruct the tube. Yet for the woman who is anxious to conceive a child, this procedure may offer the possibility that her fertility can be preserved.

THE HOSPITAL STAY

Women who suffer an ectopic pregnancy often experience a series of upsetting events. Those who don't even know that they are pregnant may be completely baffled. Some women experience mild to moderate pain for a week or longer before the ectopic pregnancy is diagnosed or the tube ruptures. For others, acute pain is the first sign of trouble. Whatever the duration or nature of the pain, the dramatic symptoms of ectopic pregnancy, including blood loss, pain, and shock, can be terrifying. As with many other women, it may have been your first serious medical ailment and likely your first brush with death.

Because the surgery was done under general anesthesia, you probably woke up, following surgery, in the recovery room, with an intravenous tube, feeling nauseated, groggy, disoriented, and in pain. You were probably heavily medicated — a period of grace. As the medication wore off, the reality struck you.

Shortly after you woke up, your husband or your doctor told you what had happened. Chances are the message you got was a minimized or understated version to avoid alarming you. Most doctors try to soften the blow at first. Your physician may have told you of the damage to your fallopian tube and what measures he took, but he may have held off discussing the implications for future pregnancies.

Several women said that their initial reaction was to feel relief that they had survived after coming so close to death. Only later did they begin to recognize what they had lost.

Following surgery, you are usually hospitalized for four to six days. Some women told us that being placed in the obstetrics area was particularly difficult. They felt that facing new mothers and babies was extremely traumatic as they realized the loss of their own child and possibly their fertility as well.

"It was worse for me emotionally than physically," Marge said. "I was on the obstetrics floor after my ectopic for five days, surrounded by happy mothers and fathers and their babies. I was particularly sensitive to seeing them because I had lost a baby and a tube. I was very distressed I might not ever have a baby as we had hoped and planned. When I got home, I could let go of my emotions, and I felt much better."

Some women felt that they were treated merely as surgical patients; their emotional needs were not met. Jane talks about her six-day hospital stay: "After surgery I was very depressed. I had known of the pregnancy less than twenty-four hours before surgery. Yet neither my doctors nor the nurses tried to get me to talk about how I was feeling. They treated it just as if it were 'another operation,' but it had a lot more meaning to me — I lost a chance to have a baby."

In all probability, as you were recovering from the surgery, you began to realize what was happening to you. In a short period of time, you experienced a life-threatening medical condition, lost a pregnancy, and lost one of your fallopian tubes. So much has happened that your head may be reeling and you may feel unable to assimilate it all. In addition, your initial feeling that you were lucky to survive has probably started to pale, and the specter of what you have lost now seems enormous.

PHYSICAL RECOVERY

Because you may have had severe pain and bleeding, perhaps even hemorrhage, and because you have had major surgery involving anesthesia and medication, physical recovery from an ectopic pregnancy can take a month, possibly longer. It is important to get a lot of rest during this time.

Most physicians prefer to do a physical examination two to three weeks following surgery. During this visit, your doctor is likely to discuss your surgery in detail and inform you of its implications for future pregnancies.

If you are having no physical problems and your incision is healing well, your physician will probably give you permission to have sexual intercourse. However, he will probably suggest that you wait until you have had three normal menstrual cycles before you attempt to become pregnant again, and that you use a mechanical method of birth control (diaphragm, condom, foam) during this time.

THE EMOTIONAL AFTERMATH

Not until you had been home for a while did the full impact of your loss strike you. You have been through a life-threatening crisis. You realize now that you could have died. You lost your pregnancy, perhaps after years of trying to conceive. You've found out that your chances for a successful pregnancy are dismal.

Added to all this is the problem that most people don't seem to understand what you're going through. You may have chosen not to tell anyone you had an ectopic pregnancy. If you told friends and relatives, it is possible that they discuss it as a surgical procedure when it is much more than that to you. They may think as long as you have "one good side," it will make little difference. But you know what your doctor has said and it scares you — your chances of having a baby are reduced and the likelihood that you will have another ectopic pregnancy is significant.

If you have other children, they may have been around during the emergency, seen you in acute pain, and not been able to understand the cause. Then you were rushed to the hospital, where you stayed for up to a week. It might have been the first time you were separated from them for this length of time. Their lives have been disrupted and it's been a traumatic period for them. Try to stay close to them so they will not feel shut out.

During the aftermath, you will probably go through times of vulnerability, bewilderment, anger, guilt, jealousy, and grief if you are like the women we counseled.

Vulnerability

It is common to feel extremely vulnerable after having an ectopic pregnancy. It may have been the first time your own life has been endangered. Your concern was not just about the baby's death, but the possibility of your own. Perhaps for the first time you had a sense of how fragile life is, how little control we have. You were lucky; they caught it in time — you didn't die and hopefully there were no complications, but the threat existed and is frightening to think of.

Bewilderment

So much has happened so quickly that you may feel completely bewildered. You were perplexed at the time when it was going on and you find that you remain puzzled as you try to sort things out.

Kathy, in her mid-twenties, expressed her confusion as follows: "I was very sad and felt a death had occurred. I felt empty and puzzled as to *why*. I comforted myself by thinking it was an early pregnancy and realizing it would have been harder to lose a baby later, as with stillbirth. I fell back on the thought that I had gotten pregnant after years of infertility. All told, my thoughts and emotions were mixed, sometimes conflicting and sometimes disturbing."

Anger

It is common to feel furious that an ectopic pregnancy happened to you. You didn't deserve it. You want a baby so badly and you are frustrated because it doesn't seem as if you'll ever have one. You realize your anger is irrational, but you feel it nonetheless. At times you are certain it was no one's fault and at other times you question whether it was. Why wasn't it discovered earlier? you ponder angrily; maybe then the damage wouldn't be so bad.

As a young secretary said: "I was 'mad at the world' at times after the loss of my pregnancy and my left tube. I was astonished at my occasional anger with some little thing that went wrong. I couldn't seem to control it. I realized I felt frustrated and didn't know what to do about it. I talked it over with my husband and he understood better why I was so irritable. I felt I needed to talk about my feelings with women who had gone through something similar, so I joined a discussion group I heard about through a friend. This helped me the most because we shared our feelings and learned we weren't neurotic — that our emotions were understandable considering the circumstances. We also helped each other cope."

Many women are disturbed by the scars of an ectopic pregnancy, both mental and physical. The physical scar is disturbing to look at, but that's not what bothers you the most. What is most upsetting is that the scar reminds you of your loss.

Blame and Guilt

You may find it hard to accept the fact that your tubal pregnancy "just happened." You feel a compulsion to find out whose fault it was and to blame someone or something for causing it.

Frequently, women blame their doctors for causing the ectopic pregnancy or for failing to diagnose it earlier. There may be times when a doctor makes a mistake, and that is unfortunate. There are many more times, however, when the tubal pregnancy could not have been diagnosed any earlier than it was.

You may blame your doctor for failing to save your tube when it was unsalvageable. Your feelings and need to place blame may get in the way of rational thought. People tend to feel angry at the doctor who "mutilated" them, as one woman termed it.

Possibly, you blame yourself for what happened. Women commonly feel guilty for things that happened in the past, thinking that "I brought it on myself." They can't forgive themselves for undergoing reconstructive surgery on their tubes despite the risks, or having contracted venereal disease years earlier. While feeling guilty serves no constructive purpose and makes you feel worse, it is difficult to let go of the idea that you are being punished for your sins.

Envy

You may envy women who are pregnant or those who have healthy children. Feeling jealous is a common reaction. It doesn't seem fair that those around you are effortlessly having babies and you envy their good luck. You may feel sad every time you see a pregnant woman or a baby, and you may find yourself consciously trying to avoid such encounters whenever possible.

Grief and Mourning

With ectopic pregnancy, there is likely to be grief and sadness on many levels. The couple mourns not only the loss of the pregnancy, but also the possibility that their fertility has been reduced. It is not unusual for a couple to have had problems with fertility prior to having an ectopic pregnancy. When this is so the couple is apt to feel a double sense of loss when a pregnancy fails because it was a long-awaited and extremely precious pregnancy.

Toby, in her early thirties, describes her terrible sense of loss following a tubal pregnancy after having difficulty conceiving. "I felt sure, after fifteen long months of anxiety, tests, and waiting, that I was finally pregnant. Then it just didn't seem possible that I was going into surgery that was to take away the baby I had prayed and longed for.

"I felt such a tremendous sense of loss and emptiness, and to top that, I felt the discomfort that follows surgery. The real depression occurred when I got home and the full impact of what happened was felt. Not only was I cheated out of a baby, but how could I ever have another one with only one fallopian tube, my husband's low sperm count, and my irregular ovulation?

"To me, the odds were overwhelmingly against me. For weeks I'd find myself crying for that lost baby that I was never given a chance to feel or know."

For Toby and many others, losing a pregnancy was extremely painful. They experienced many of the emotions common to early pregnancy loss described in Part I. In addition, their feelings of grief were often compounded by feelings about the loss or reduction of fertility which resulted from the ectopic pregnancy.

With ectopic pregnancy you may grieve less for the actual baby, since you knew you were pregnant for such a short time, if you knew at all, than for the lost opportunity, your lost fertility. Sandy describes her delayed grief: "Since I didn't even know I was pregnant, the whole thing seemed like emergency surgery and not much more. Then, later, it hit me that I had lost a baby. However, I felt the most anxiety when it sank in that my chances of having a successful pregnancy in the future were much lower."

Meredith had similar feelings and commented on the impact her tubal pregnancy had on her life. "I only knew for a few days that I was pregnant so I didn't have time to get very excited. But we had been trying to have a baby for eighteen months, so I did get excited for a few days and was terribly disappointed the way things turned out. I felt very badly in the months that followed the loss. It is only lately that I have been gradually improving; there is still much depression and despair. Occasionally, I have had mild suicidal impulses. We have wanted a child for so long and we have no idea what the future holds. With one tube gone, I know my chances of getting pregnant are less, and I have an increased chance of another ectopic pregnancy. That absolutely terrifies me. I grew up thinking of pregnancy as a wonderful time, and now that has been ruined."

After an ectopic pregnancy it is necessary to heal both physically and emotionally. Fortunately the process of physical recovery is almost always uneventful and is usually accomplished within a month or two. Emotional recovery tends to occur more gradually as one comes to terms with what has happened, and as one assesses what one has lost and what is still possible.

Many women have found that the support and understanding of friends and family were invaluable in helping them along this road. If it is at all possible, talk to others who share your experience. They have a special knowledge of what you have been through. These conversations should convince you that you are not alone, that your feelings are comprehensible, and that other women have felt the way you have and have managed to pick up the pieces of their lives and go on. This can be both a solace and an inspiration.

They have made it and you can. The natural course of grief is one of gradual healing. There are also things you can do to speed your recovery. Anything that reconnects you to life helps: seeing friends, working, socializing, to name a few. Do not be discouraged if at first it takes an effort to do these things. Each step along the way should be easier than the one before it.

THE HUSBAND'S EXPERIENCE

Your husband is likely to have many of the same emotional reactions to the ectopic pregnancy as you have had. He, too, will be affected by the pregnancy loss because, like you, he wanted a child, and no doubt he shares your sadness at learning that his chances of becoming a parent are diminished.

Yet your husband's concerns about losing the pregnancy and about decreased fertility were probably overshadowed by his fear of losing you. When you pulled through, the fact that you survived was utmost in his mind. He may seem less upset than you are about losing the baby. It's not that he didn't want the baby; it's just that he was terribly worried about you and feels grateful that you are all right.

Most men develop an attachment to their unborn child later in the pregnancy than their wives do. With ectopic pregnancy, this attachment may not have developed at all, since the pregnancy terminated so early. In fact, your husband may not have even known you were pregnant. Within the span of a few hours he may have been confronted with the news that you were pregnant, that you were being rushed to the operating room for emergency surgery, and that you would lose the pregnancy. That was a great deal for him to handle all at once. He, too, was probably shocked, and like you, he had to deal with feelings of bewilderment and pain.

Men and women generally perceive pregnancy differently, so chances are that your husband coped with the pregnancy loss, surgery, and implications for fertility in a different way than you did. For a better understanding of how the experience differs for husbands and wives, we suggest you read chapter 8, on the marital relationship.

WHAT CAUSES ECTOPIC PREGNANCY?

In about half the cases of ectopic pregnancy, no cause is found. The most common causes of interference with the progress of the fertilized ovum are damage to the tube from chronic pelvic inflammatory disease (usually secondary to gonorrhea and, rarely, associated with postabortion infection), previous pelvic surgery, or a prior ectopic pregnancy or reconstructive surgery (tuboplasty).

Other conditions thought to be causes are developmental abnormalities of the tube such as excessive length, diverticula involving outpouching of the tube and kinking, obstruction from sources outside the tube itself, and hormonal factors that affect the transport of the egg through the tube. At the present time there is some evidence that women who have used an IUD (intrauterine device) in the past have a higher incidence of ectopic pregnancy than might otherwise be expected. If a woman has an IUD in place at the time of conception there is a 3 to 9 percent risk that the pregnancy will implant ectopically; this is a significant increase over the usual rate of occurrence. Similarly, "progestin-only" oral contraceptives, known as the minipill appear to be associated with a fivefold increase in ectopic pregnancy in the population of women who conceive while taking them. There is no increased risk for women taking combination (estrogen-progesterone) oral contraceptives.

Pregnancy is rare in those who take the "morning after" pill, but when it does occur there is a tenfold increase in the incidence of ectopic pregnancy. There is also an association between ectopic pregnancy and certain male factors: both an abnormal sperm count and a high percentage of abnormal sperm seem to contribute to the risk.

GETTING ON WITH YOUR LIFE

It was bad enough to lose the baby after trying hard to get pregnant, but the final blow came when your doctor told you that there was even more to be concerned about. If it was your first ectopic pregnancy and you have one tube left, your chance of getting pregnant again may be diminished. Only 50 percent of women conceive after having had an ectopic pregnancy. In addition, there is an increased chance that there may be something wrong with your remaining tube, for whatever caused the problem with your first tube (such as obstruction secondary to pelvic inflammatory disease, tubal surgery, or infection) may also have affected your remaining tube. Unhappily, the woman who has suffered one ectopic pregnancy has an increased risk, 7 to 12 percent, depending on the study, of having a second.

If your tube had previously been removed (this may be your second ectopic pregnancy) or you know it is badly damaged or malformed, it is highly possible that your fertility may be grossly impaired or completely absent.

When the initial shock has worn off and you are feeling better physically, you can begin putting things into perspective. One thing is clear: becoming a parent will be no simple matter. You have a long, hard road ahead of you. For a while, you'll need to assimilate what has happened and you will need to grieve. When you feel ready, you will deal with what to do next: get another medical opinion, try to conceive again, undergo reconstructive surgery, adopt.

It is best to enter into the decision-making process after you understand your medical condition completely — what you lost and what you have left. It is then that you can look at your alternatives and consider which is best for you.

(1) If you have potential fertility, you must decide whether to try to get pregnant again. In doing so, you may be risking another ectopic pregnancy, however.

(2) If you have had conservative surgery that salvaged your damaged tube, or if you have tubal obstruction on the opposite side, you need to decide if you want to undergo reconstructive surgery. When successful, this surgery should improve your chances of conceiving. However, one unfortunate consequence of the surgery in some women, is that scarring resulting from the tubal surgery may increase the possibility that another ectopic pregnancy may occur.

(3) If you are infertile, as a consequence of having lost both tubes or because your tubal damage is too extensive for reconstructive surgery to be helpful, the choices that remain to you are adoption or childlessness.

For those who are potentially fertile and decide to try again, it still remains to be seen whether or not Nature will do her part. When conception does not occur, there are many stresses to contend with. Among these may be diagnostic tests to assess whether or not you have an open fallopian tube or tubes, basal body temperature charts to maximize your chances of getting pregnant, months of eager anticipation followed by crushing disappointment, and maybe even reconstructive surgery to repair a damaged tube. If conception occurs quickly, one hurdle is passed, and the anxious waiting begins. Only when it has been definitely established that the pregnancy is intrauterine is it possible to breathe a sigh of relief.

If your problem is not one of uncertain fertility, but one of definite sterility, this must be dealt with. Under the best of circumstances, it is extremely difficult to make peace with the loss of your capacity to reproduce. However, when you feel robbed of your fertility by an accident of nature, or by the unforeseen consequences of your own actions, the loss may be even more difficult to accept. When an ectopic pregnancy causes infertility, there is more than physical damage to contend with: your sense of wholeness is also impaired, and your psychological well-being is threatened. The dual nature of the assault complicates the grieving process. Not only must one mourn the loss of fertility; the loss of one's body wholeness must be coped with, too.

Despite the fact that your options are clear, you may feel confused and unable to make a decision. This is a common reaction after ectopic pregnancy. After all, this has been a major life crisis and it may take a long time before you recover. You have had to come to terms with the issue of death — no simple task for *anyone*. Often, people who have been traumatized by a recent brush with death have trouble in making decisions. It may help you to know that one day everything will fall into place and you will find your choice clear.

One Woman's Story

We were sitting in a cafe with friends on a Sunday afternoon when I felt the first pains. My heart sank — cramps, I thought, even though my temperature hadn't dropped at all that morning. I gazed at the chart of my basal temperature several times every day like some ancient priestess trying to divine the future by observing the flight of birds. I had been taking my temperature for four months as part of the fertility workup my gynecologist was conducting. For a year now I had greeted each new cycle with the hope that this time I would become pregnant, and every time the menstrual flow began I experienced increasing disappointment and frustration. This time I had watched the days pass, ritually acknowledged every morning on the chart — 28, 29, 30. . . . I became more hopeful and more excited. And now, I was sitting, talking with friends, outwardly calm and cheerful, but inwardly terribly sad. I didn't feel any flow beginning, but that was usual for me. Cramps could signal the beginning of the menstrual flow several hours before it began in earnest. But I was very surprised and confused when I got home several hours later and still found no flow. But the cramps persisted.

Monday morning the thermometer registered 99°. The cramps and the continuing absence of menstrual flow had me puzzled. I so much wanted to believe that the temperature chart meant that I was pregnant, but my body seemed to be telling me otherwise. I debated inwardly for a while, and then called my doctor. It turned out that he was out of town attending a conference, and I was put through to the physician who was taking his cases. I described my situation and current symptoms, but the doctor didn't think they warranted an office visit.

Tuesday morning my temperature was over 99°. Since 99° was the highest number on the chart, I drew the line up above the chart to approximately where I thought the next degree markings would go. The chart was still my oracle, but not a very interpretable one. I could never get my temperature line to go in the neat ups and downs of the illustration. Staying up late, having a glass of wine, or sleeping in late all would affect the temperature reading.

I was not working at the time. I had quit my job half because I wanted time off and half because I optimistically expected to be pregnant. I offered my help at a little theater some friends of ours were starting up. On that Tuesday morning I still had cramps and was glad I was scheduled to work as rehearsal assistant because I thought that activity would take my mind off my discomfort and distract me from my growing uneasiness about the meaning of the pain. Halfway through the rehearsal the pain became so intense that I couldn't sit upright in my chair. I apologetically told a friend that I had to leave. She took one look at my face, white and beaded with sweat, and whisked me off home.

Of the number of things I learned during the whole frightening process of the ectopic pregnancy, one of the most important for me has been how to present myself to physicians when I need medical help. I grew up in a family in which stoicism and the unflinching endurance of pain were main values. I accepted without question that the appropriate behavior, no matter how intense the pain, was calmly to describe the problem to the doctor and wait for him to help me. My regular gynecologist knew me fairly well, and he recognized this feature of my character (we talked about it after the whole experience was over). But the physician taking his place had no such background knowledge of me, and he based his judgments on his experience with his patients in general.

This time, when I called, the doctor said to come right in, and he squeezed in time between two scheduled patients to see me. I came into the examination room clutching my temperature chart in my hand and holding myself carefully upright. I calmly described my symptoms to him, and then he examined me. Then he said it was unclear what was going on. I might be pregnant, but it was too soon to tell. Sometimes pregnancy produced puzzling symptoms, like pain, but it couldn't be an ectopic pregnancy, because I didn't have enough pain. And what, I inquired quietly, constituted enough pain? Pain so intense that women scream and roll around, he said.

I was dumbfounded. I could not begin to explain that I could not imagine a circumstance that would cause me to act like that. When I was a teenager, my mother fell down while hiking and broke her leg in two places. My father carried her to a fire road, and from there she was evacuated by jeep. She never screamed or rolled around, although it was clear that she was in considerable pain. The pain the doctor was describing was clearly outside my realm of experience, and my pain did not qualify as a major symptom. As I left the doctor's office I was aware of being deeply embarrassed. I had committed an unforgivable sin — I had acted like a hysterical female.

My husband had taken me to my appointment, and as we drove home I passed on the doctor's assurance that I was all right because I didn't have enough pain for it to be an ectopic pregnancy. He didn't know exactly what an ectopic pregnancy was, so when we got home I drew him a picture of the ovaries, tubes, and uterus. He was relieved that that was not the problem, but since he could see that I was still uncomfortable, he asked if maybe I should go see our internist. The covering doctor had suggested that my symptoms might not be the result of a gynecological problem, but I was still so embarrassed at crying wolf that I refused to consult another physician.

I passed the rest of that day and night in a fog of ambiguity. What did the pain mean? Was I pregnant and about to miscarry? Was I just having a difficult period? Did I have a strange form of appendicitis in which the pain appeared on the left side instead of the right? I tried to get my mind off my pain and my worry. But no sooner would I succeed in distracting myself than I would find my attention going back to my abdomen. Had the pain diminished? Yes, it did seem less than before; no, wait a minute, that was quite a strong twinge — and on and on.

Except for my doctor, no one knew that we were trying to have a baby. At first, I had just wanted to present my friends and family with a fait accompli. I had thought that I would be pregnant within a few months of deciding I wanted to be. Then, as the months drew on and nothing happened, I became even more reticent about telling anyone. I feared there was something wrong with me — something very deeply wrong — and I didn't want anyone to know. So now during the days of ambiguity I had no one, except my husband, with whom to share my fear and my longing. My husband was, as always, my mainstay. He took care of me, and kept track of how I was feeling. But even he did not understand my deep longing for a baby, and so could not share my emotions. Not until the doctor finally gave a definite diagnosis and I was being wheeled into surgery did he grasp the meaning of the loss.

Wednesday morning, my temperature went up another notch. I was half joyful, half despairing. In the months before, the line on the chart had taken that long plunge that indicated the onset of menstruation, and my hopes had plunged with my temperature. So part of me still hoped that I might be pregnant, and everything would be all right. But another part of my mind thought that at least if my temperature dropped, I would have some clarity about what was going on. I almost began to hope that it would drop, that the bleeding would start and I would have some resolution.

During the morning the pain became more and more intense. I must have picked up the phone fifteen times to call the doctor, but each time I put it down again. How much pain was enough? I didn't want to risk feeling like a fool again. Finally, around midday I was overwhelmed by a sharp, intense, sickening pain. This had to be enough pain. I lay on the sofa, too ill even to get to the telephone. Then the pain subsided. I felt better. Good thing I hadn't called the doctor, I thought, or he'd really have me pegged as a hypochondriac.

My husband called in the middle of the afternoon to see how I was doing, and was greatly relieved when I told him that I had had a lot of pain in the morning, but it had now all gone away. Although I didn't know it at the time, that intense pain was the tube "blowing" (to use the doctor's word). The tiny

embryo that had somehow implanted in my tube and found enough nour-
ishment to grow had burst the fallopian tube. So I was happy in my igno-
rance that afternoon, and cheerfully went about doing chores I had neglected
for the past few days, not knowing that all the while I was bleeding internally
and that in a short time I was about to experience "enough" pain.

The first twinges definitely felt like cramps. I went upstairs and took my
temperature again, even though it was late afternoon. I still had a low-grade
fever. Could I have some infection that was causing the fever and masking
the usual drop before my period? I was again swamped in ambiguity.

I felt some nausea by evening and didn't eat much dinner. I left the table
before my husband had finished eating, and went upstairs to lie down. He
soon followed me worriedly into our bedroom. In the next hours, as the pain
increased and I found it impossible to read or distract myself in any way, he
kept pacing around and checking on me. He tried to get me to call the doctor.
I didn't want to bother the doctor at home, I told him. When he said he was
going to call, I yelled at him, and then cried. We called the doctor.

As before, I spoke to the doctor calmly and quietly. I described my symptoms
in detail. He prescribed codeine, and my husband went to an all-night
pharmacy to get it. I awaited his return impatiently. At last, something to
relieve the pain. I might then begin to be able to think straight and extricate
myself from this web of fear and pain.

The codeine upset my stomach. I stumbled into the bathroom to vomit, and
realized that I felt very faint. My husband half carried me back to the
bedroom. I could neither stand nor sit up without blacking out. I lay on the
bed writhing in pain and moaning. My husband called the doctor back and
described what was going on. I was too ill to talk. My husband had no
personal rules about telling the doctor in unemotional tones what was going
on. He conveyed his worry and concern. The doctor said he would meet us
at the hospital.

The trip to the hospital had all the elements of slapstick comedy. Had I not
been so sick I would surely have protested. I live two blocks from the hospital.
But since I could neither stand nor walk, and since my husband couldn't
carry me down the stairs to the car, he called an ambulance. As it turned out,
their stretcher couldn't fit down our stairs, so the men ended up carrying me.
The ambulance attendant called me "honey" and regaled me with stories of
other people he had transported that night (the one right before me had a
gunshot wound). My husband rode in the front and gave the driver direc-
tions — he didn't know how to get to the hospital.

Once we arrived at the emergency room, there began what seemed like an endless series of examinations. By this time, the accumulated blood in the abdominal cavity was causing spasms in all the abdominal muscles, and the pressure of the blood on the diaphragm caused referred pain in my upper chest. The merest touch could set off these incredibly painful spasms, and it seemed as if people never stopped poking, prodding, pushing, and feeling. My husband squeezed my hand and stroked my head while I cried and begged them to stop. Finally I heard myself screaming.

At long last, they stopped and I was left alone with my husband while they awaited the results of some blood tests. I felt sure that I was dying, and I wanted to tell my husband how much he meant to me, and what a good life we had had together. I was searching for the words, but he was already on another tack. If the doctor didn't come up with anything definite, he said, he was going to call our internist. They weren't sure it was a gynecological problem anyway. The doctor came back in and said that the tests were inconclusive and that they were going to put me under observation. The doctor's announcement sent me into despair. This was it, I thought; they were just going to watch me die. My husband went out into the hall with the doctor and came back to tell me that they had called our internist.

It wasn't my regular internist who arrived, though, but one of his associates, whom I had never met. He was a young man who immediately dispensed with any pretense at a bedside manner. I later forgave him because he quickly got to the root of the matter, but at the time it was a little disconcerting. The other doctors had been very kind and concerned, apologizing for hurting me. This one began with a series of accusatory questions — what drugs had I been taking, how much did I drink? He acted as if he knew that I was a dope-fiend alcoholic. His certainty convinced even me. I confessed that I did usually have a glass of wine with dinner.

When he began to examine me, I could feel another painful spasm starting. I knew that if he touched me, it would start up an agonizing series of spasms. As he reached out his hand, I grabbed him by the wrist with all the strength I could muster. He gave me a startled look. I could see that I had scared him. It must be an unwritten rule that the doctor touches the patient, but the patient does not touch the doctor.

Then he was in charge of the situation again. His examination was quick and incredibly gentle — not what his manner had led me to expect. Then he took my blood pressure. They must have taken my blood pressure a hundred times since I had been admitted. He left the blood pressure cuff on my arm and told me to sit up. I told him that I couldn't, that I passed out when I sat up. He just put his arm behind me and hauled me into a sitting position and took my blood pressure again while everything slowly went black before my eyes. He lowered me again. Then he placed his stethoscope on my abdomen and with two fingers pushed down as far as he could and let go suddenly. I could see my abdomen rise first on the right side, then on the left, as the fluid inside sloshed back and forth.

These two tests seemed to clinch it for him. He went into a huddle with the gynecologist, and then the quiet room was bustling with activity. No one told me anything. Suddenly, I was swept over with the most exquisite sensation of relief. It was as if someone had taken a magical eraser and wiped the pain from my body. They had just given me intravenous Demerol. They had their diagnosis; they no longer needed my pain as a guide. Then the final test — a needle through the abdominal wall to see if there was blood in the abdominal cavity. There was.

Things happened quickly after that. My husband had stayed by my side throughout the ordeal. At the doors to the operating room we had to part. I panicked. I fought against the drug-induced euphoria. Now I had to say something, because I might not make it through. "I love you, I love you" was all I could think to say. He kissed me, and then I was wheeled into the operating room.

The anesthesiologist was immediately by my side, introducing himself and asking if I were allergic to any drugs. All the while he was rigging up an apparatus, and introducing another needle into my arm. I could see that I would be out cold in a matter of seconds. I asked where the doctor was, and pleaded with the anesthesiologist to wait before he put me out. I was told the doctor was preparing for surgery and would be along in a minute, but they had to go ahead with their preparations.

The anesthesiologist began to inject the sodium pentothal. "Give him a message from me, please," I begged. The doctor slowed down his injection. I was beginning to fade. "Tell him to be conservative," and then I was out. I went down fighting for control of the situation, and desperately afraid that the doctor might not try to salvage what he could of my reproductive organs. No one had told me what the surgery would consist of — I thought I might wake up to find I had had a hysterectomy.

The next few days run together for me. They are not a blur, but rather a series of vivid scenes. From this point on, everything that had to do with pregnancy or babies was very highly charged for me. The loss of the embryo and the loss of the tube made me even more obsessed with becoming pregnant, but initially I was sunk in grief. I found reminders everywhere.

I woke up in the intensive care unit because the recovery room was not yet open. I was definitely in the way there, and I heard grumbling around me. They sent a maternity nurse down to take care of me. Once in my hospital room, I found that one of my roommates had had a hysterectomy. The other was an eighteen-year-old girl who already had two children and was in the hospital for an abortion.

My husband came late in the morning. He had stayed outside the operating room until the surgery was completed. He had talked to the doctor, and then gone home to sleep. He told me he had been overwhelmed when he realized that there had been a tiny baby — part of him and part of me. Up till then, our efforts at pregnancy had somehow seemed theoretical to him. But now, too late, he grasped the reality, and the loss seemed awful.

Calling my parents and telling them was very hard. My mother had been planning to visit, and she advanced her time of arrival to coincide with my getting out of the hospital. I'll never forget the shocked look on her face when she saw me get out of the car on my homecoming day. Acting in the family tradition, I had played down my illness to her. Her face told me better than any mirror how ghastly I looked.

The doctors had decided not to transfuse me because they had recently had problems with the current supply of blood — people had been contracting hepatitis. So I was supplied with iron pills and a diet that included red meat twice a day. The anemia, however, was one of the hardest things I had to deal with. It took me a couple of months to build myself up again, and the inability to do anything without sweating, panting, and feeling exhausted added greatly to my depression.

I quickly got back into the fertility workup, though. The doctor advised a certain period of time for recovery from surgery, and then I was again taking my temperature every morning, and having intercourse on prescribed days at prescribed times. I cross-examined the doctor on the probability of a second ectopic, and we set out a plan for how to deal with it if I even suspected I might be having a second one. I found out that there is an association between infertility and ectopic pregnancies. But I was also assured that many women bear full-term babies after having an ectopic pregnancy. I lived with the hope.

Six months later the doctor recommended that I see a specialist. He summed up his findings and said that the evidence was inconclusive as to what was wrong. His best guess was that something was not quite right with the remaining tube. On the other hand, he said, it might be something else too subtle for his tests to pick up. I told the doctor that I needed a break, and he agreed that this might be a good thing.

It is one of the ironic conditions of life that the anxiety to become pregnant can act to interfere with impregnation. I hoped that if I could get away from the daily fascination of the temperature chart and the monthly timing of intercourse, I might achieve through relaxation what I couldn't through science. By this time my relationship with my husband was under strain. I was obsessed with becoming pregnant, and our sexual life had lost all spontaneity. When we visited friends of ours who had a new baby, I would be fine during the visit, then sob all the way home in the car.

In addition, I was haunted by memories of the ectopic pregnancy. I couldn't shake the horrifying memories of those days of pain. It could hit me almost anytime, but particularly in that time of going to sleep, when the conscious guards are down, I would suddenly be thrown back into the nightmare, reliving it second by second. Then I would turn my face into the pillow and cry. My husband would hold me and try to comfort me. He didn't understand what was going on, but he was infinitely patient with me.

So I called a halt to the further pursuit of infertility consultations, and I entered graduate school to prepare myself for a new career. Too much idle time was grist for the mill of depression. I threw myself into my work, and derived considerable satisfaction from it and from the new friends I made. But nearly a year and a half after the ectopic pregnancy I realized that I was still reliving the terror. This was not healthy, I decided, and I started seeing a therapist. She helped me tremendously. I dealt with and got rid of the waking nightmare. It became an experience of the past, instead of one I relived constantly in the present. And I dealt with my own deep fears about there being something wrong with me because I wasn't able to become pregnant.

My time spent in therapy was a tremendous liberation for me. Freed from the shackles of fear and bad feelings about myself, I could begin to think in a new light about having a child. I was no longer obsessed with pregnancy. I wanted a child very, very much, but my whole sense of myself as being all right did not depend upon it.

I went to see the specialist my gynecologist recommended. He concurred with my physician. There was most likely something wrong with my remaining tube. Surgery might be able to correct it. If it could be surgically cor-

rected, he would give me a 30 percent chance of pregnancy. I was not impressed by the odds. I cried all the way home.

I talked it over with my husband, and thought about it a lot myself. If I had the surgery and if the tube could be repaired, there was still no guarantee of pregnancy. I remembered the months of the reign of the thermometer and the scheduled intercourse, the waiting anxiously every thirty days, the depression and the despair.

One weekend while I was still debating with myself about the surgery, I had an experience that made up my mind for me. I was gardening in my front yard. A little girl who lives several houses away was trying to learn to ride her two-wheeler. She could go a few yards before she fell over. She fell near where I was weeding, and I helped her up and then spent some time holding her bicycle straight and pushing her while she strove to get the feeling of balance. All the while, as usually happened whenever I was around children, I was filled with an intense longing to have children of my own to love and care for and help learn to ride bicycles. Then it hit me. I looked at the little girl and realized — I could love this child. She doesn't have my genes or my husband's. She doesn't look like either of us, but I could love her as if she were my own. Here I had been spending all my time thinking only of pregnancy. What I wanted was a baby.

That was the turning point. What happened next is truly another story. Briefly, I'll say that we pursued an independent adoption, and within a year we were holding a beautiful, healthy baby boy in our arms and bringing him home. As I write this now, we are on the eve of our day in court when the adoption will become legal. We are very pleased to have all the legal proceedings complete, but from the moment we first held him in our arms we knew he was our baby.

It took four weeks from conception for the embryo to burst the fallopian tube. It took four years from the ectopic pregnancy to reach the decision to adopt. I now have accepted the loss of the baby that might have been and the loss of my own reproductive function, but I know that, for me, it took a long time.

5 ❧

Prenatal Testing — When a Problem Is Discovered

Not so very long ago pregnancy was a mysterious process. Once initiated, it remained out of one's control until the time of delivery. In the last decade, however, techniques for examining the genetic, metabolic, and structural makeup of the fetus have been developed, and this technology has made it possible to diagnose a wide variety of abnormalities before a child is born. Although prenatal diagnostic techniques are most often used to screen for chromosomal abnormalities in fetuses carried by women over thirty-five (the most common of these being Down syndrome, or trisomy 21), scientists are also capable of identifying many other genetic and metabolic abnormalities. Research is currently being carried out that will allow scientists to map out the human genome and dramatically expand our ability to diagnose genetic disorders.

In the United States most pregnant women who receive prenatal care will undergo some type of prenatal screening. As a result, some couples will be spared the anguish of carrying a fetus with severe abnormalities to term, while others will be able to avoid producing a child with life-threatening or -impairing disorders. A fortunate majority will be able to relax and enjoy their pregnancy, secure in the knowledge that prenatal testing did not detect an abnormality.

Our ability to diagnose an ever-increasing number of conditions prenatally stands to have a profound effect not only on individual lives but on society as a whole. There are ethical issues to be considered, such as how to apportion limited resources and how to decide what level of risk an individual must have in order to be tested. How does one determine which conditions are serious enough to justify terminating the pregnancy, and who should make the decision — parents, physicians, or society? Should parents be informed about all genetic and metabolic abnormalities — even those with minor or unknown consequences and those that are diagnosed incidentally? What effect will our ability to selectively terminate pregnancy have on the way in which those who choose *not* to terminate are treated, on our attitudes about handicapped people, and on the way that those born with prenatally diagnosable disorders will feel about themselves?

THE EMOTIONAL IMPACT OF PRENATAL DIAGNOSIS

The choice of whether or not to have prenatal diagnosis may affect your pregnancy experience in many ways. In general, the earlier in pregnancy a test can be performed, the earlier results will be obtained, and the less invasive it is, the less emotional trauma it will cause.

Parents who perceive that there is a significant risk that the fetus could be affected with a disorder often delay forming an attachment to it. This has been variously described as "trying to think of it as a condition rather than a pregnancy," "not letting yourself think about the baby inside," and "not permitting yourself to expect anything or to plan for the future." Many women report that they felt numb until they learned that the fetus was normal; only then could they let themselves feel happy and excited. Others report feeling incredibly anxious and unable to seek comfort because they did not want anyone else to know that they were pregnant until they themselves knew whether they would be carrying the pregnancy to term. Those who were most affected by such common symptoms of early pregnancy as nausea and vomiting found it hardest to push thoughts about the pregnancy out of their consciousness.

Many women who choose amniocentesis find themselves on "emotional hold" until somewhere around the twentieth week of pregnancy. Half of their pregnancy will be over before they know what the outcome of the testing is. Those who get good news feel enormous relief and are eager to enjoy what is left of their pregnancy. However, even when the news is good, it is common for women to feel that the whole experience has been difficult. Many women prefer not to tell others that they are pregnant until the test results are back. This means wearing clothing that hides the fact that they are pregnant and not letting friends, family, coworkers, or children know. For many this is a lonely, frightening time, made more so by the absence of the comfort and support that would normally be available to them if others in their world knew what they were going through. When you wait to have an amniocentesis and then must wait still longer to get the results, time passes very slowly. Life can feel unreal, as if you were suspended on a planet where you are the only visitor. It is painful to think about the pregnancy, and deadening not to. Looking back on her pregnancy, a thirty-eight-year-old woman reported that "Waiting wasn't a lot of fun. At that point the baby was moving a lot so I couldn't avoid thinking about it." Since amniocentesis is most often done between the sixteenth and twentieth week of gestation, it is likely that "quickening" will occur before the results are in. Quickening, the experiencing of first feeling the baby move, generally happens at eighteen to twenty weeks and is thought to represent the point in the pregnancy when women experience the fetus as a separate being and form an increased attachment to it.

As the time for the amniocentesis approaches, most women find themselves feeling increasingly anxious. Even those who have been through the procedure before and know that it is quite simple and painless may find themselves focusing much of their anxiety on the procedure itself. Displacing anxiety is one way of getting through a difficult time or event, but this method of coping is not without its painful aspects.

Most women find the amniocentesis itself to be much less traumatic than they had anticipated. A common reaction is to feel that your anticipatory anxiety was much greater than the procedure actually warranted. In contrast, most people find the ultrasound scan, which is used to identify the location of the fetus and placenta, much more thrilling than they had thought it would be. It is possible to see a recognizable form after as little as sixteen weeks of gestation, especially if the various parts of the baby are pointed out. The psychological impact of the ultrasound is considerable for many couples: it presents undeniable evidence that you are indeed carrying a child, despite your best efforts to keep from thinking about it. It is not unusual for couples to feel an increase in attachment to the pregnancy after seeing the baby on ultrasound. It is also common to experience conflicting feelings — both pleasure at seeing your future child and anxiety at the thought that there could be something significantly wrong with it.

The period between having the amniocentesis and obtaining the results is an especially difficult one for most people. Seeing the baby on ultrasound makes it harder to avoid thinking about it. Hope and fear creep in when you are least expecting them. As the time nears when the results will be available, anxiety tends to increase. It becomes even more difficult to wait: you want to know that all is well and live in dread that your worst fears may come true. Every time the phone rings, panic sets in. In addition to feeling anxious, women report having frightening thoughts and nightmares about what may be wrong with the baby; many also feel emotionally fragile and vulnerable and may be easily moved to tears.

SCREENING TECHNIQUES

Ultrasound

Ultrasound visualization of the fetus is a noninvasive procedure in which intermittent high-frequency sound waves are passed through the mother's abdominal wall, where they are absorbed differently by fetal tissues of different densities and then echoed back to a display screen where they generate an image of the fetus. This technique is used to establish the gestational age of the fetus; to assess whether its size and growth are normal; to verify that the pregnancy is intrauterine; to demonstrate the presence of a fetal heartbeat; to identify any fetal and placental abnormalities; and to determine whether the amount of amniotic fluid that surrounds the fetus is normal.

A thirty-three-year-old first-time mother who requested an ultrasound "because I wasn't a candidate for amniocentesis and I wanted to know if everything was normal" described her experience as follows: "We had the ultrasound done at nineteen weeks. The technician was very quiet. My husband knew something was wrong before I did. The doctor came in and told us that the baby had a serious heart defect. It was a total blow. We finally had gotten pregnant and we expected to have a perfect child — this news meant for sure this wasn't to be." While this woman's experience is unusual in that she requested that an ultrasound be done to detect Down syndrome, a purpose for which it is not well suited, it is not unusual for structural abnormalities such as this one to be diagnosed during a routine ultrasound examination.

Maternal Serum Alpha-Fetoprotein Screening Test

Another commonly employed prenatal diagnostic technique is that of screening for alpha fetoprotein (AFP), a substance produced by the fetus and identifiable in the mother's body.

At specific times in a pregnancy, measurement of the AFP level in the mother's blood or in the amniotic fluid may help to identify the presence or absence of certain abnormalities in the fetus, the most common of these being a developmental abnormality of the brain or spinal cord called an open neural tube defect. The maternal serum alpha-fetoprotein (or MSAFP) screening test is usually done between the sixteenth and eighteenth weeks of pregnancy. Of every 1,000 women screened, 950 will have normal results.

If the initial screening test shows abnormally high levels of MSAFP, ultrasound examination will enable your physician to determine whether the results were abnormal because the gestational age was incorrectly estimated, because there are multiple fetuses, or because an abnormality of the brain or spinal cord is, in fact, present. Amniocentesis is then performed to either rule out or confirm the presence of a neural tube defect.

Recent research has indicated that abnormally low MSAFP levels may also be helpful in identifying fetuses with Down syndrome. In such cases, ultrasound examination can be utilized to demonstrate whether any of the structural features that may be suggestive of Down syndrome are present. Amniocentesis may then establish the diagnosis.

In normal fetal development, the tube that forms the brain and spinal cord closes completely by four weeks; if this fails to occur, the fetus will have a neural tube defect. Eight to 9 percent of the time, the neural tube defect will be closed — that is, covered by skin — and thus not detectable by MSAFP screening. In the United States one or two of every thousand babies will have a neural tube defect. The two most common types of neural tube defects are anencephaly, a severe disorder of the skull and brain that almost always results in a stillbirth or death soon after birth, and spina bifida, a malformation in which the spinal column fails to completely enclose the spinal cord. Spina bifida may be associated with a range of clinical outcomes: some children with the disorder may develop normally and have little or no physical or mental impairment, while others may experience varied degrees of paralysis, loss of bowel and bladder control, loss of sensation in the legs, hydrocephalus (water on the brain), and mental retardation. A recent study has revealed that when spina bifida is diagnosed prenatally, parents choose to terminate the pregnancy 90 percent of the time. When anencephaly, which is incompatible with life, is identified prenatally, most parents will choose to terminate the pregnancy.

DIAGNOSING GENETIC DISORDERS

At the present time, universal genetic testing is not done for a number of reasons: because for most women the potential benefit of the procedure is less than the risk involved; because laboratory space is limited; and because the cost of screening every pregnant woman for every identifiable abnormality would be prohibitive. Genetic testing is instead reserved for the population at greatest risk: women over thirty-five; those who have some family history of a genetic disorder, a neural tube defect, or inherited skeletal, metabolic, or hematologic disease; those who have previously had a child with one of the above conditions; and those who have been identified as carriers of a genetic abnormality by a variety of screening techniques or assessed as being at risk because they belong to a particular ethnic group. The majority of couples who seek prenatal genetic testing do so because advanced maternal age has put them at increased risk of producing a child with Down syndrome. Down syndrome is a chromosomal disorder that causes mental retardation and a characteristic physical appearance and is associated with an increased incidence of heart defects (30 to 50 percent) and gastrointestinal tract abnormalities (8 to 12 percent). Techniques that allow physicians to examine the genetic material of the fetus include amniocentesis and chorionic villus sampling.

Amniocentesis

Amniocentesis is a technique whereby a sample of amniotic fluid is obtained by inserting a needle through the mother's abdomen and into the amniotic sac that surrounds the fetus. Ultrasound is used to guide the placement of the needle so that the risk to both the placenta and the fetus is minimized. Amniocentesis is usually done between the sixteenth and the eighteenth weeks of pregnancy because at that point it is possible to obtain a sufficient amount of amniotic fluid to perform the necessary diagnostic tests. The feasibility of performing amniocentesis around the twelfth week of pregnancy is currently being assessed.

Once the amniotic fluid is withdrawn, it is taken to the laboratory, where fetal cells are removed from the fluid. These cells are grown until they have multiplied sufficiently so that chromosomal studies can be done. The entire process can take anywhere from seven to twenty-one days.

Chorionic Villus Sampling (CVS)

In this technique, a sampling of cells is taken from the chorionic villus, either transabdominally or through the cervix. The chorionic villi are located outside the amniotic sac but inside the uterus: they form a layer of fetal membranes through which fluid is exchanged between mother and fetus. Because they develop out of the union of egg and sperm, they are composed of the same genetic material as the fetus itself and so can be used in the same way as cells obtained through amniocentesis. The advantage of chorionic villus sampling (or CVS) is that it can be done during the first trimester of pregnancy, permitting an earlier termination of the pregnancy when necessary. The disadvantages of this procedure are a miscarriage rate that is five times higher than that associated with amniocentesis and a lower degree of accuracy. In addition, there have been some recent reports of damage to the fetus resulting from this sampling process.

New Diagnostic Tests

New techniques are currently being developed that will allow genetic disorders to be diagnosed earlier in pregnancy than is now possible. One of the most promising of these is a procedure in which a sampling of blood is taken from the mother early in her pregnancy. The small number of fetal cells that have passed into the maternal circulation are then separated out for analysis.

Another experimental innovation is a rapid amniocentesis technique known as fluorescent in-situ hybridization, or FISH. In conventional amniocentesis, cells cannot be examined for abnormalities until they have been grown in the laboratory, a process that normally takes one to three weeks. Using the new FISH technique, scientists have been able to examine the nucleus of cells immediately after obtaining them by amniocentesis, by means of fluorescent probes or artificially constructed chromosome segments that selectively attach themselves to those areas of the fetal chromosomes where defects are most likely to be present.

DECIDING ON PRENATAL GENETIC TESTING

In deciding whether or not to have an amniocentesis or chorionic villus sampling, you will need to weigh the costs against the potential benefits. On the cost side of the ledger are the risk of trauma to the fetus, the umbilical cord, the placenta, or maternal tissues; the danger of infection; and the chance of premature labor and/or miscarriage caused by the procedure. (Amniocentesis done with ultrasound visualization by an experienced practitioner has been shown to be quite safe: under these conditions the rate of pregnancy loss is less than 1 in 200.) Also on the cost side are the expense of the procedure (often covered by health insurance for those deemed to be at risk) and the impact the choice may have on your pregnancy experience.

Although the risk of producing a child with Down syndrome and/or other chromosomal abnormalities increases gradually over a woman's reproductive life span, a sharp rise in incidence occurs at around age thirty-five (see table 5.1). Women over thirty-five are considered to be at the greatest risk and thus to derive the maximum benefit from amniocentesis. The effect of paternal age is to increase or decrease the maternal age-related risk by 1 percent for every year older or younger the father is than the mother. When the fetal chromosomal material is examined for Down syndrome or other suspected abnormalities, the overall chromosomal structure of the fetus is also assessed, and other chromosomal abnormalities may be diagnosed.

Table 5.1: Risk of Having a Live-Born Child with Down Syndrome

Maternal Age		Risk of Down Syndrome
20	one in . . .	1,923
21		1,695
22		1,538
23		1,408
24		1,299
25		1,205
26		1,124
27		1,053
28		990
29		935
30		885
31		826
32		725
33		592
34		465
35		365
36		287
37		225
38		177
39		139
40		109
41		85
42		67
43		53
44		41
45		32
46		25
47		20
48		16
49		12

(Permission to use this table of incidence was granted by V. Dimitriev and P. L. Oelwein, eds., *Advances in Down Syndrome* [Special Child Publications, 1988].)

DECIDING WHAT TO DO

Most couples who choose to have an amniocentesis or chorionic villus sampling have decided in advance that if a genetic disorder is diagnosed they will terminate the pregnancy. However, this is not always the case. Some couples treat the choice to have an amniocentesis and the choice to terminate the pregnancy as two independent decisions. Andrea, age forty, felt strongly about having an amniocentesis: "I knew I wanted to have an amnio because I wanted to be prepared for whatever we would have to deal with. The decision about whether or not we would terminate was put on hold until we knew what the results of the amnio were and had a chance to learn all we could about the condition our child had."

It is not unusual for couples who have decided in advance what course of action they will take if an abnormality is diagnosed to find themselves rethinking their decision once the information is in. Even those who come to the same decision they originally made find it helpful to go through the process again. One of the basic tenets of genetic counseling is that no one really knows what he or she will do until he or she is faced with a diagnosis and must make a decision about what course of action to take.

One factor that affects the decision-making process is whether or not both partners agree on the decision. Parents may differ in their willingness to take risks, in their attachment to the pregnancy, in their desire for a child, in their religious beliefs, or in their feelings about living with a handicapped child. In order for a joint decision to be made, each partner must be willing to appreciate the other's point of view as well as to explain his or her own. Reaching a decision together may involve allowing your partner the time he or she needs to weigh the alternatives, or giving you both time to talk about how different choices may affect your lives individually and as a family.

Decision making is particularly traumatic for couples who are faced with a situation that is not clear-cut, either because the abnormality is not adequately described in the medical literature or because it may be associated with a spectrum of clinical manifestations. Individuals differ markedly in terms of what level of risk or handicap they are able to deal with. "For some people a 15 percent risk that there may be a problem is more than they can live with, while for others an 85 percent chance that the baby will be all right is an acceptable level of risk," says Dr. Wayne Miller, of the Prenatal Diagnostic Center of Lexington, Massachusetts.

The level of uncertainty that an individual or couple can tolerate or is willing to accept is affected by many factors. Underlying character structure determines both the individual's ability to tolerate ambiguity and his or her intrinsic optimism or pessimism. Previous life experiences are also important: those of us who have experienced painful losses are often less willing to take a risk than those who have been more fortunate. Whether a couple has other children, whether or not the pregnancy was planned, and how attached the parents are to the pregnancy may all have an influence on what decision is made. Couples who have a history of infertility and for whom this is a "premium pregnancy" — perhaps achieved after years of trying or through one of a variety of financially, physically, and psychologically costly assisted reproductive technological procedures — may be more accepting of risk than those who have had no previous difficulty in conceiving.

The impact of receiving a diagnosis of a genetic, metabolic, or structural abnormality seems to be different for those who perceive themselves to be at risk — whether because they have been previously identified as carriers, because they have had an affected child, or because they have a known family history — than for those who do not consider themselves at risk. The two groups probably form different levels of attachment to the pregnancy, with those fearing poor outcomes tending to postpone the process of attachment even more than is usual for those who choose prenatal diagnosis. In the event that the fetus is diagnosed as affected, those with a known family history are more likely to receive social support for a decision to terminate because their choice will in all likelihood be better understood and thus more sympathetically received.

Factors Complicating Your Decision

Couples who learn that their fetus has the same disorder as another child, a close friend or relative, or the mother or father must deal with complex feelings. It is often hard to separate your feelings about a person you love who has a specific problem from your decision about whether or not to bring a child with the same disorder into the world. For example, parents who already have a child with Down syndrome or spina bifida need to be clear that the decision they make is independent of their love for their existing child. Instead of thinking about your love for your first child and whether you are glad that you had him or her, it is helpful to focus on whether or not you have the resources, stamina, and ability to cope with a second handicapped child. In families where there is a known history of a genetic disorder, parents may find the decision to terminate particularly painful. Similarly, when one or both partners have been identified as carriers, they may feel guilty and responsible and may fear that their spouse consciously or unconsciously blames them. Although this is most often not so, it can make the decision-making process a potential mine field for both partners.

Another difficult situation is that in which one fetus in a multiple pregnancy is found to be abnormal. Parents must decide whether to continue the pregnancy without intervention, whether to terminate the entire pregnancy, or whether to choose to selectively terminate one fetus. The dilemma they face is a difficult one: the decision to continue without intervention means bringing a child with major problems into their lives, and the decision to selectively terminate means taking the risk that the unaffected fetus or fetuses may not survive the trauma of the termination procedure. A similar dilemma confronts parents who are found to be carrying three or more healthy fetuses, often as a result of infertility treatment. Since multiple pregnancies are high-risk in regard to the incidence of both fetal death and prematurity, an assessment must be made as to whether the risk of selective termination is greater than that of not intervening. In both of these situations parents have a difficult psychological road to navigate: the decision to risk the life of a healthy fetus is always an agonizing one. In addition, a baffling onslaught of feelings may engulf the parent who is faced with simultaneously mourning the child who has died and rejoicing in the child or children who have survived.

MAKING THE CHOICE TO END
THE PREGNANCY

Just as you cannot predict how you will feel until you are actually *in* a situation, it is equally impossible to adequately prepare yourself for bad news. However hard you may have tried to put your feelings on hold, and as much as you may have attempted not to invest in the pregnancy or even to think about it very much, the news that something is wrong comes as a powerful blow. As with all painful losses, you will probably feel some combination of numbness and disbelief at first. This is one of the ways we protect ourselves from being totally overwhelmed. Gradually you will absorb the reality of what has happened, and grief will replace the numbness.

It is usually a good idea not to make a decision about what to do immediately. Although you may have anticipated the outcome and may be clear about what you want to do, try to give yourself some time. You will want to discuss your options with your spouse. Your physician is available should you want to talk, as are other doctors and counselors trained in human genetics. A geneticist or genetic counselor can help you understand what the problem is, what spectrum of difficulties you can anticipate, what effect these may have on your child's life and on your own, and what other factors you should consider in making your decision. You may also want to arrange a consultation with a pediatric specialist who can outline the clinical picture as well as tell you whether treatment is available and what it is likely to entail. Assimilating complex medical information and deciding what course of action to take can be difficult under any circumstance; at a time when you are in a state of shock and feeling overwhelmed, it may be all you can do to think straight, much less make a critical decision in a short space of time.

If you make the decision to terminate the pregnancy, you will suffer a unique type of pregnancy loss. Reactions to this loss vary and may include feelings of sadness, anger, guilt, uncertainty, and isolation. A critical difference between this kind of loss and a miscarriage is that you have made a deliberate decision to end the pregnancy. You may be shocked to discover that you are capable of choosing to terminate. It is a particularly difficult time for those whose decision goes against their personal or religious values. Those who choose to terminate often do so with mixed feelings: on the one hand, this probably was a wanted pregnancy; on the other hand, it may be a relief to be able to choose not to produce a severely damaged child. Experiencing such contradictory feelings as grief and relief simultaneously can be emotionally exhausting. Even those who are sure that they have made the right decision and those who know that the "choice" to terminate was more illusory than real may feel guilty. Deciding against life under any circumstances is a painful burden and an uncomfortable responsibility. To make matters worse, couples sometimes feel that they are out of sync with each other in terms of what their predominant feelings are at any given moment. Sometimes this causes one or both partners to feel emotionally abandoned.

One factor that influences how parents experience the loss of a fetus with genetic difficulties has to do with their fantasies. One couple discovered that they were having difficulty appreciating each other's reaction to the decision to terminate a pregnancy in which the fetus had a serious genetic disorder because they were mourning different children. The husband had formed a vision in his mind of a child with the particular difficulties their child would have had, and it was with sadness but also with relief that he experienced the loss of this child. In contrast, his wife's attachment was to the perfect baby she had imagined in the months before the results of the testing were known. Her grief was for this ideal child and thus was much more painful and long-lasting than her husband's.

As with all types of pregnancy loss, the experience may be different for each parent. A woman often forms an attachment to her pregnancy earlier than her husband does, which tends to make the loss both more intensely painful and longer-lasting for her. In addition, since the child was carried in her body, she is likely to feel more involved in the pregnancy. The decision to terminate likewise involves her more directly, as it is she who must go through either a dilation and evacuation procedure (or D and E) or the induction of labor and delivery. Some partners find that the experience of dealing with bad news, making a decision together, and supporting each other in a time of grief brings them closer together. Others feel isolated and unable to connect. One partner may want to talk, while the other may prefer to handle his or her grief privately; one may want to let others know what has happened, while the other may feel that no one else should know; one may want to join a support group or go for counseling, and the other may not want to. Here as in all aspects of marriage it helps to remember that you are two separate people, with different needs and different coping styles. If you allow your spouse to do things his or her way, understand his or her experience, and support his or her efforts to cope, and if your spouse does likewise, you are less likely to feel alienated from each other.

Even when grief is shared, each person must cope with the onslaught of his or her own painful feelings. Initially the pain is overwhelming, all-encompassing, and seemingly without end. You may find yourself angry that this has happened to you; you may feel guilty, even though you know you did nothing to cause the problem; or you may blame yourself or your spouse, even though you know it is irrational for you to do so. Most people find themselves wondering why this terrible thing has happened to them, to their child, to their family. Families who have had a previously affected child may find that old feelings of anger, disappointment, and grief are reawakened, and these may compound the pain of the current loss. Most people feel sad; some cry easily and often; others feel low, flat, and locked-in. Feelings of sadness normally continue for several months or longer. This can be particularly difficult when you are trying to keep what has happened a secret. The task of carrying on in a normal manner while your life feels like it is falling apart may be all but impossible to pull off. You may find that grief affects many aspects of your life, draining your energy, making it impossible for you to take pleasure in anything, making you feel hopeless and helpless, isolating you so that you can't relate, or releasing a torrent of words and feelings that won't stop. Sometimes self-esteem is affected as well: you may feel "genetically inferior" if you are the carrier of a genetic disorder, or you may feel inadequate for not producing a healthy child like everyone else.

Many couples find that their sexual relationship also suffers. Depression dampens and sometimes extinguishes sexual desire, and the problem may be compounded by feelings of low self-esteem, a postpartum hormonal state, and the fact that sexual relations remind you of your loss and make you feel vulnerable.

TERMINATING THE PREGNANCY

Once the decision has been made to terminate the pregnancy, most women want to get it over with as soon as possible. However, it is not always feasible to arrange an elective procedure immediately; sometimes it is necessary to wait several days before a termination can be scheduled. Lydia felt that "It was very hard to wait the three days for the abortion. I kept saying to the baby, Don't move. I don't want to feel you move anymore."

Second-trimester terminations are performed either in a special clinic that is equipped to do late abortions or in a hospital. The two most common methods of terminating a pregnancy around the twentieth week of gestation are dilation and evacuation (D and E) or induction of labor using saline or prostaglandins. The former procedure is preferred by some physicians because it spares the woman the necessity of going through labor. The woman is either heavily sedated or given general anesthesia and then the cervix is dilated and the fetus is extracted from the uterus. As the fetus is usually too large at this stage of pregnancy to be removed whole, D and E can be an upsetting procedure for both the medical staff and the couple, who may be left with disturbing thoughts about what went on.

Those physicians who prefer to induce labor feel that it causes less trauma to the woman's body. They also believe that it is psychologically sounder to allow couples to complete the process as naturally as possible. Whenever labor is artificially induced, the resultant contractions tend to be strong and very uncomfortable; however, in the case of a second-trimester termination, it is possible to use medication to help control the pain. After delivery, couples who wish to can see the fetus. Most couples who choose this option feel that having an actual visual memory makes it easier for them to grieve the loss.

When a pregnancy is terminated in the second trimester, the body behaves as if a premature delivery has occurred. This means that you are likely to experience both breast engorgement and mood changes as your body readjusts its reproductive hormone levels (for details, see chapter 3).

WHETHER OR NOT TO TELL

Whether or not to let others know is a decision that everyone who chooses to terminate a pregnancy must deal with. This decision tends to be complex on many different levels. First, you may be feeling uncertain and guilty about choosing to terminate. If this is the case, you may also tend to assume that others will feel about you the way you feel about yourself. Second, this issue is one that evokes deep feelings in many people. You can never be sure what you are going to tap into when you tell someone else about the choice you have made. Most people's worst fear is that others will be critical of their decision, judge them, or think they are a terrible person.

If people know that you were pregnant, one option is to present the loss as a naturally occurring miscarriage. Another choice is to select whom you choose to tell the truth to. It is not necessary to tell all to everyone; acquaintances, coworkers, and neighbors need only know that you lost a pregnancy. If there are friends or family members to whom you feel particularly close, you may want to tell them what happened. If you stop to consider your relationships with different people, you will know whom you trust and whom you want to share the truth with. One advantage of sharing is that the support that friends and family can give may be enormously helpful. Those who choose to tell people they trust tend to be amazed by the understanding and support they receive.

If you have kept your pregnancy a secret, the choice is not so much *what* to tell but *whether* to tell. In this situation you need to decide which way of handling things will be best for you. It is important for you to recognize that you have been through a painful loss and a traumatic experience and that you need to keep your own best interests in mind and take care of yourself as well as you can.

One option that many people find helpful is joining a support group made up of individuals and couples who have been through a similar experience. Such a group can offer you a safe haven in which to talk freely with others who understand. The process of talking about a traumatic experience and allowing yourself to feel the pain can be healing, and it is helpful to give and receive understanding and support. For further information on support groups, see the resource section beginning on page 243.

One Woman's Story

At the time of the abortion, I was sixteen weeks pregnant. When I was eleven weeks pregnant, I had seen an ultrasound image of our baby floating inside my uterus, its heart beating. By the fourteenth week, I could feel the baby move inside me, faintly but distinctly, and I looked pregnant. Inspired by my new shape, my husband and I had taken to calling the baby Bump. At my age, the risk of a first-trimester miscarriage was much greater than the risk of Down syndrome. Having come this far, we began to believe that we had beaten the odds and were going to have a child at last.

Then the results of the amniocentesis came. In the moment I heard my doctor saying he had bad news, all of the beauty and hope of what had seemed like a flourishing pregnancy were destroyed. It was like being told of the sudden, unexpected death of a loved one. In reality, though, this would be a death that my husband and I would have to choose. I was totally unprepared for everything I experienced after that telephone call.

My husband and I wanted that pregnancy very much. I was forty-three years old, and Daniel was forty-five. It is a second marriage for both of us. Although we each have one child from our prior marriages, we felt we were missing important parts of the experience of being parents: my son spends part of every week with his father, and Daniel sees his daughter only on alternate weekends, for alternate school vacations, and for a long vacation in the summer. Moreover, we wanted to be parents together. It is just not the same thing to share the parenting of a child who is not the natural child of one of you. We wanted a child whom we could both love with the unequivocal love of a natural parent and who, for better or worse, would be an expression of both of us.

And it had not been easy getting as far as we had with that pregnancy, which was the second we had had together. Our first step was to get over the fear that our marriage would also end in divorce — the fear that if we had a child, we would wind up inflicting pain on the child (as we had on our other children) as we pulled apart from each other. Next came the waiting to get pregnant. We tried to get pregnant for eight months without success. My doctor then suggested that I have a hystero-salpingogram, which showed everything to be normal. Two months later, I conceived with Daniel for the first time, but I was afraid to believe it.

I had had two miscarriages before the birth of my son and the miscarriage statistics for someone my age were discouraging. I did what I could to protect myself from becoming invested in this first pregnancy with Daniel, especially because I didn't "feel" pregnant. My pregnancy that went to term from the beginning felt very different from the pregnancies that miscarried. This one didn't feel right. In my eighth week, as I stood in the kitchen washing the dishes, I felt a sudden flow of warm fluid down my legs. I knew immediately what it meant. The amniotic sac had broken, signaling the beginning of a miscarriage and the end of a pregnancy. I didn't have the sense of disbelief I had had with the earlier miscarriages — I knew to anticipate that it might happen. But the sense of failure and sadness was the same — or maybe worse, because this loss brought back all the old pain that was still inside me.

The next day, after a night of heavy bleeding and cramps, I saw my doctor. His examination was inconclusive. I had an ultrasound the following day. Having bled so much, I expected to see a picture of an empty uterus. Instead, what I saw on the ultrasound screen was an image of a little living thing and a weakly beating heart. The radiologist said the fetus didn't look viable, but she couldn't be sure. She told me that I would just have to wait and see what happened. I bled persistently for the next week and then went for another ultrasound. Everything that had been in the uterus had disappeared. I had had a complete miscarriage. My doctor instructed me to wait for one period; after that I could try again.

Miraculously, after waiting the prescribed time, I became pregnant in my next cycle. I tried not to think about it. I did my best to go through each day as if there were nothing unusual going on. But this time, though, things were different. I began to feel really pregnant. By the fourth or fifth week, I was extremely fatigued and nauseous. After another week of so, I was nauseous both in the morning and at night, and I didn't feel so well in between, either. It became a struggle to get through each day, to go to work and take care of my son. Feeling so sick, I couldn't help but pay attention to this pregnancy. By taking hold of my body so vigorously, the pregnancy overwhelmed my defenses and forced me to think about the life inside me. Moreover, the sicker

I felt, the more confident I became that I was not going to miscarry and that the pregnancy was normal. During my first appointment with my doctor, at eight weeks, he told me that everything looked right on target. We scheduled an appointment for a week later to talk about prenatal diagnostic testing.

As I look back on it, I realize that Daniel and I went to that appointment with the attitude that it was just a formality — a sort of courtesy that the doctor was extending to us in case we were not as educated as we thought we were about prenatal testing. The discussion was matter-of-fact. The doctor described the two types of prenatal diagnostic test procedures (amniocentesis and chorionic villus sampling, which no one in Providence, Rhode Island, then performed but which was available at the Yale–New Haven Medical Center in Connecticut) and the defects that the tests can identify. He then explained Down syndrome, the most common genetic defect in babies of older women, and illustrated his explanation by drawing a little diagram of how the extra chromosome appears in the twenty-third chromosomal pair. We talked about the odds — the likelihood of our having a problem — and about how long it would take to get the test results. I asked the scary question about what type of procedure I would have to have if we terminated the pregnancy. We were assured that it would probably be "just" a D and C procedure performed on an outpatient basis, and that I would not have to go through labor and a vaginal delivery. However, the doctor did say that he did not do second-trimester D and C's and would therefore have to refer me to someone else if such a procedure was needed.

Sometime in the course of our meeting, the doctor said that of course we shouldn't bother having a prenatal test unless we were prepared to terminate the pregnancy if the tests disclosed a problem. Nothing that we were told during that "counseling" session helped or encouraged us to come to terms with what that simple statement meant. We never talked about how Down syndrome might affect the life of the individual child or the child's parents. (What is the nature of the defect, and how severe is it? Is there any way to know how impaired a particular baby will be?) We were told that amniocentesis might be less likely to trigger a miscarriage than chorionic villus sampling but that the test must be performed later in the pregnancy and that results took longer to get. Having said that we were inclined to choose amniocentesis because of our fear of miscarriage, we were not told how much difference the extra weeks would mean in terms of the development of the pregnancy and our attachment to the baby. We never talked about how devastating an experience it is to choose to terminate a pregnancy, even if you are convinced that it is better not to bring a child afflicted with Down syndrome into the world. There was no acknowledgment that in addition to facing the pain associated with losing any pregnancy, we had to be prepared to decide whether to end the life of a baby whom we would love and whom we desperately wanted.

It may be that given the odds, it is better not to discuss these things with every women who is considering prenatal testing, but rather to wait until you know that there is a problem. By talking about them with everyone, you inflict worry needlessly on women who will never have to face the decision of whether to abort. But if you wait until the test results are in, you deprive the parents of the opportunity to prepare themselves in advance. Once the bad news comes, the pain is so great that it is hard to think clearly.

It was another three weeks or so before the amniocentesis was performed. I continued to count the days — each day was a day when I overcame the risk of miscarriage and came closer to being able to love my baby with all my heart and to fantasize freely about what life would be like with another child. During that three-week period, Daniel and I took a vacation on St. Bart's, in the Caribbean. Even in that paradise, the days went by slowly and my energies were consumed by the effort to deal with the nausea and the pleasure-dread of the pregnancy. After we returned, I continued to throw up so forcefully that my doctor suggested an ultrasound, which I know was primarily for the purpose of reassuring me that things were all right. And indeed they were. On that day, in my eleventh week, I saw our baby on the ultrasound screen. The baby looked like a baby. It was squirming around and sucking its thumb. I could see that it had beautiful, delicate hands and a lovely fragile profile. The technician remarked that it was a beautiful baby. Lying on the ultrasound table, I cried with joy.

Up to this time we had told only my sister and one other couple, our dearest friends, about the pregnancy. Seeing the ultrasound picture made the pregnancy so real to us that Daniel and I began to discuss whether to tell the children and the rest of our family. As we debated the issue, the decision was taken out of our hands. One evening my ten-year-old son came up to me, put his hand on my belly, and asked, "Mom, are you pregnant?" Although we did not tell my son that evening, because we thought it was important for the children to hear the news together, we prepared to tell them on the next weekend when the whole family could be together.

Like the ultrasound picture, telling the children transformed our experi-

ence of the pregnancy. Within the family, we began to talk about it a lot. The children expressed their feelings about it (many of them surprisingly negative), and I, for the first time, could talk about how I was feeling. The children then had their telling to do. Even though we explained that it was possible that we might not be able to have this baby — I might miscarry, and we had to have a test to find out if the baby was healthy — the children had to tell their other parents and their friends about this impending change in their lives. It also became clear that people other than my son thought I looked pregnant. The rumors were flying in the office. Daniel and I began to share the news with a wider circle of friends and with people with whom we worked closely. As we made the pregnancy "public," the fact that we were going to have a child became a larger and larger part of our lives. Nervously, I shopped for a few items of elastic-waisted clothing.

The day I had the amniocentesis was a cold, gray day in February, punctuated by heavy rain. We arrived on time for our appointment, at the same office where my earlier ultrasounds had been done, and sat anxiously in the waiting room for almost an hour while my doctor finished a delivery at the hospital. Finally we were called into one of the ultrasound rooms. The technician set up the ultrasound and my doctor and the radiologist arrived. As the procedure was being performed, the doctor described what he was doing: deciding where to insert the needle, administering the topical antiseptic, inserting the needle ("Now this may be a little painful. You may experience some cramping"), drawing out the amniotic fluid, withdrawing the needle. In between these comments my doctor and the radiologist talked animatedly about other cases they were both involved in, and they rushed off together as soon as the procedure was finished. Although it had been more painful than I'd expected, and I felt faint for some time afterward, there was an anticlimactic quality to the whole experience. The professionals handled it with the same dispatch as a Pap smear. I had expected them to tell us what they could discern about the normality of the baby from the ultrasound image, but they didn't. No one said that the baby was beautiful. We drove the test sample to the laboratory ourselves (a precaution the doctor follows to minimize the risk of the sample's being mixed up with someone else's) and I went home in the pouring rain and feel asleep, exhausted.

In truth, I don't remember much about how I felt as I waited for the test results. Perhaps it is because the quality of the waiting was so similar to what I had experienced from the beginning of the pregnancy. From the beginning

I had been waiting to know that things were all right. I was told that the results might not be available for two weeks but that it was possible that the laboratory would have something to report in ten or eleven days.

On the tenth day, at about ten in the morning, I called the lab to find out when they expected to have the results. The woman at the lab responded that they had already reported some results to my doctor and that I should get in touch with him. It was then that my anxiety became unbearable: there was something in the woman's voice that frightened me. There was no joy in her voice, as I imagined there would be if there had been good news to tell, and no words of reassurance. I immediately called my doctor's office. The line was busy, as it often was, and it remained busy all morning as I hit the "Repeat/ Dial" feature on my office telephone over and over again. When I finally got through, I got the answering-machine message saying that the office was closed for lunch but that I could have the doctor paged at the hospital if it was an emergency. At that point I told my husband, who works in the next office building, about my call to the lab.

With our denial mechanisms telling us that nothing could be wrong, my husband and I went to a scheduled lunch meeting. At its conclusion we returned immediately to my office and tried to reach my doctor again. When we reached the answering machine again, I called the hospital and asked for the doctor to be paged.

When my doctor got on the phone and heard who it was, his first words were, "Did the laboratory tell you already?" This question and the tone of his voice made my stomach turn and my insides tense. Somehow, though, it still took my breath away when he proceeded to say that there was a problem. All of the cells that had grown out so far showed an extra chromosome in the twenty-third pair. As he put it, it was "classic trisomy." The lab had called him that morning, but he had been waiting until evening to call and tell us so that we could hear the news when we were at home. He said how sorry he was and added that we were lucky that there was a way to find out about these things in advance. We didn't feel lucky. He then explained that he would call the physician who would perform the abortion, whom he described as being very kind and gentle, and that doctor would call me back to make an appointment.

After the phone call, Daniel held me in his arms as I cried. I wanted to scream, to wail, to pound on the walls, to do something to let out the pain. At the same time, I couldn't believe what we had heard. I couldn't believe that this had happened to us, that I was that one woman in thirty-two over the age of forty-three who has a Down syndrome child. And I was filled with despair. I was certain that we would never have a child together. I was too old, and there was obviously something wrong with me — all of the miscarriages and then a Down syndrome child. I couldn't possibly go through all this again. I felt the loss of the baby inside me, and the loss of all hope.

I don't recall that my doctor asked us whether we wanted to terminate the pregnancy. He just assumed we did, and so did I. In fact, I wanted to terminate the pregnancy immediately. I think that if my doctor had said during that phone call that I could go straight to the hospital and do it, I would have done it. It seemed that the only way to do something about the incredible pain of knowing there was something wrong with the baby was to get rid of the pregnancy as quickly as possible. I couldn't wait for my doctor to make the arrangements for me. Before leaving my office, I called the office of the doctor to whom I had been referred, explained the situation, and asked for an appointment. I was told that the doctor could perform the abortion three days later. I was devastated. Three days seemed like forever to wait — to have to live with a child inside me whom I loved and was preparing to kill. There was no alternative, however. We had to wait. We scheduled three appointments with the new doctor: one to come in and talk, one the afternoon before the abortion, during which certain preliminary procedures would be taken care of, and one for the abortion itself.

Then Daniel and I went home. It was a Monday. I would not return to the office for two weeks. I cried as we drove home and for the rest of that day. My son was at his father's that afternoon and for dinner, so Daniel and I were alone until evening. I don't remember being able to do anything other than grieve on that day. It was like being in shock. Daniel and I didn't even talk much. We just held each other. I couldn't stop crying. When my son came home, we told him that we had gotten the results of the prenatal test, that there was a problem with the baby, and that we were going to terminate the pregnancy. He had many questions, which we tried to answer. He asked factual questions that were easy to talk about: what exactly is Down syndrome, would the baby be retarded, how do they perform the abortion, and so on. It was obvious to him that you would not choose to have a Down syndrome child, and raised in our pro-choice family, he did not question but that it was a woman's right to have an abortion. At the end of the conversation he confided that even though he knew we were very sad, he was relieved that we were not going to have the baby that threatened to upset his life again. While I was pleased he could share his feelings with me, his sentiments deepened my grief. It seemed then that Daniel and I were isolated in our sadness, with only each other to hold on to.

I awoke Tuesday morning unable to believe what was happening to us and dreading the day ahead of me. The most unbearable aspect of the whole thing was having to continue living with the feeling of the baby inside me, with the feeling of being so pregnant. Notwithstanding all the mental cautions, I had come to love that feeling and the promise it held. Once a source of constant pleasure, this feeling had become the source of the greatest distress. Daniel stayed home with me that day and waited for our two o'clock appointment with the doctor.

We were seen first by the doctor's assistant. She collected the necessary information from us and then explained the nature of the abortion procedure that the doctor would perform. As she spoke, I cried. It sounded so much worse than I had expected. I hadn't known that the procedure would have to be performed in the hospital; my previous, postmiscarriage D and C's had been done in the doctor's office. I hadn't known that the procedure would actually begin the day before, with the insertion into my cervix of a seaweed-like substance that would begin to dilate my cervix as it expanded with the moisture from my body, causing cramping during the night. I hadn't known that there really was no effective local anesthesia to relieve the pain of the uterine contractions that would be stimulated by the abortion procedure. But worst of all, I had never imagined that because I would be treated in a day surgery unit, Daniel couldn't be with me during the abortion. He could have been with me if the child were being born, but not if it was going to die.

Suddenly I became angry. I was angry at my doctor for minimizing or failing to warn us about the difficulties we were facing, and for abandoning us to this stranger we were talking to. When things were going well, he was there; now that things were awful, he was gone. I was angry at the nurse who was spewing information at us but was unable to look us in the eye or utter one sincerely sympathetic word. I was angry at the hospital for not permitting husbands to be with their wives at such a needy time. And finally, I was angry at having a baby with "a problem." In ways that I still don't understand, I think that the anger was the precursor to reaching beyond my defenses and coping mechanisms and finally — but not until the eve of the abortion — confronting the decision we were making. We spent a few minutes with the doctor, went to the hospital for the necessary preadmission laboratory work, drove to my internist's office to obtain the written referral form authorizing the procedure, as required by my health plan (and without which the hospital would not treat me), and then went home.

The next day was another day of waiting. Daniel went to work and I tried to fill the time doing mindless errands. My greatest fear was that someone would look at me and make some remark about the fact that I was pregnant, and I would respond with a torrent of tears. Just left to my own thoughts, I wept on and off throughout the day. Now I was also afraid of having the abortion. I was afraid of the pain. I had given birth to my son without anesthesia, so I knew I could deal with the pain of childbirth, but I didn't know if I could cope with the pain of the abortion. As they teach you in natural childbirth classes, part of the technique of dealing with pain is to focus your mind on something else. For me, in childbirth, that something else was the child about to be born. Now there was nothing positive to focus on — the pain was all there was. And Daniel wouldn't be there with me to support me with his love. The fear fed my desire just to have the whole thing behind me.

At four o'clock we arrived for our second appointment with the doctor and were taken into an examining room to wait. Seeking a distraction, I picked up a copy of one of the magazines in the room. Among other articles, it featured a story about a young person with Down syndrome who was starring in a television series about a family with a Down syndrome child. Feeling that it was something like an act of God that I had found this at this moment, and saying nothing to my husband, I began to read the article. I stopped when the doctor came into the room, and got up on the table to proceed with what Daniel and I had decided to do without ever even discussing it. The insertion of the seaweed produced a tolerable level of discomfort. Relieved to have that first step over with, Daniel and I went home again, stopping on the way to rent an armful of movies, on the assumption that either the cramping or our anxiety might keep us from sleeping that night.

It was not until we got home that night before the abortion that the floodgates of my feelings about what was happening really opened. Until then, the pervasive need I have to be in control of my life had prevented it. As with so much else in my life, I had responded to this crisis by trying to gain control over it — by taking the initiative in making the appointment with the doctor rather than letting my obstetrician do it, and by becoming absorbed in the arrangements and the procedures and even in the plans we had to take the family on a ski vacation the following week, plans we had made when we assumed that I would be pregnant and unable to ski. I had not let myself think about why I would choose not to have a Down syndrome baby, or about what it meant to choose not to have a baby at this point in a pregnancy. Now I thought about the Down syndrome child who was acting on television, I thought about a friend's Down syndrome child, and I thought about how much I wanted to have a child of our own. I also let myself think about the living person inside me, who, if he lived, might be a television actor or just a loving, friendly child like our friend's child. I wondered if it was too late to turn back — if the abortion was already so far progressed that we couldn't turn back. Then I thought about what having such a child would mean for Daniel and me and our other children. I thought about my strengths and weaknesses as a person and my ability and willingness to care for a disabled child. It wasn't until then that I felt I had made a choice to have the abortion. Until then I had been operating on assumptions: of course we would have a prenatal test so that we could avoid the tragedy of having a Down syndrome child or a child with other defects detectable before birth, and of course we would exercise the hard-fought-for right of women to have control over their bodies by choosing to have an abortion. As Daniel and I talked that night, for the first time (and the only time since I have known him), he cried. He cried for the death of our baby. I cried with him. Until then I had been saying I would never go through all of this again — no more pregnancies, no more losses, no more pain. It was just too much. But that night, as we grieved for our baby and for our loss, we talked about trying again. We shared the feeling that we would redeem Bump's life if we had the courage and the good fortune to have another child. Nevertheless, I have never felt a greater sorrow than I did that night.

I slept fitfully through the night, awakened by cramps. They were not as severe as I had feared, and had I not been so overwrought, I don't believe they would have disturbed my sleep. At seven o'clock on Thursday morning, we drove through the snow to the hospital. When we arrived at the special day surgery unit, which is used predominantly for abortions, I was grateful to be placed in the care of a mature, intelligent, and sympathetic nurse who would stay with me throughout the morning. Her character and the kindness with which she cared for me, together with Daniel's love, made all the difference to me.

The nurse brought us into an area of the unit that had hospital beds separated by curtain walls, and we were given one of these spaces for our home base. I changed into a hospital johnny. The nurse promptly started an

IV and gave me a sedative. She then sat with us to answer questions and tried to make us as comfortable as possible about what was going to happen that morning. Unlike the nurse at the doctor's office, she asked questions about who we were and about our family. She talked with us about how difficult a thing it was that we were doing. She had a special ability to be both cheerfully encouraging and empathetic with our grief.

The doctor arrived on schedule, and the nurse wheeled my bed into the operating room in the unit. I was then moved onto an operating table and required to put my feet into stirrups, assuming the familiar position for an ob/gyn exam. Sheets were draped over my knees so that, thankfully, I could not see what the doctor was doing. My nurse stood at my side holding my hand and explaining what was going on. A mixture of codeine and Valium was fed to me through my IV tube, and the doctor injected a local anesthesia into my cervix. Even with the medication, my anxiety level was sky-high. The doctor then removed the fetus from my uterus using surgical instruments, and then a vacuum, and then the instruments again. I experienced a great deal of pain, and I screamed and cried as I had never done during childbirth. With no emotional resources left to be brave or in control, I asked for more codeine and Valium. Then it was over. The procedure itself took only about twenty minutes, and I was in the operating room for no more than forty-five minutes. I did not ask whether the baby was a girl or a boy, nor did I ask what the doctor would do with the baby's remains. I didn't want to know.

I was then wheeled back to my curtained cubicle and to Daniel. He was so relieved to see that I was all right and, like me, to know that it was over. Afterward I was glad he had not been in the operating room with me. One of the hardest things about the whole process for Daniel was being helpless: there was no way he could take any of the physical burdens from me. It would have been excruciating for him to watch me suffer as I did during the abortion. He kissed my hands and face. The love I felt for Daniel was really the only remedy for the pain.

Less than two hours after the abortion, most of the effects of the medication had worn off, I had eaten for the first time since dinner the night before, and we were permitted to go home. It was early afternoon, and my son was still at school. I went upstairs to bed and fell asleep immediately. I got up to have dinner, helped with homework and bedtime, and went gratefully back to bed for the night.

It was a great relief to have the abortion behind me. The fear and anxiety were gone. The feeling of the baby inside me was gone. There was just emptiness. I rested the next day (it was now Friday), reading in bed and sleeping and talking to family and friends on the telephone. And both by necessity and by desire, I began to turn back to the normal activities and demands of life. That evening Daniel's daughter would arrive for the February school vacation, and as we had planned, we would go to Maine for the week to ski, delaying our departure until Sunday to give me an extra day to recover.

The physical recovery was easy. Other than being tired, I had no physical problems after the abortion. Although I was warned that I might have heavy bleeding and that I should avoid strenuous physical activity (like skiing) for at least a week because it might cause heavy bleeding, I began to ski with the family on Monday of the vacation week and skiied all week without any ill effect. Emotionally, however, I was far from recovered. As I had been warned, my milk came in the day after the abortion. That set me back a lot. And the milk was only an external sign of the enormous hormonal changes that were going on in my body. I continued to feel very vulnerable and weepy during the whole week we were away. On the third day of skiing, I remember getting off a chair lift at the top of the mountain and without warning beginning to sob and shake. I skiied back to our condominium and got into bed. Maybe I was doing too much, but I think it would have been worse if I had done less. I felt fortunate to have the distraction of being in a beautiful place with happy children, even if I couldn't keep up with everyone else's energy and spirits.

It was worse when we came home and I went back to work. I was wearied by the questions and the explanations. To most people, we simply said that we had "lost" the baby. For a long time I was upset by all the reminders of Bump — I hadn't realized how much mental planning I had done around the baby. I had expected to have a maternity leave from work; now work seemed tedious, and I wanted to escape from it. The baby's due date was July 25, so we had expected not to take our usual two-week August vacation trip. As the months passed after the abortion, although I am generally the family vacation planner, I couldn't bring myself to plan that trip, and Daniel finally had to step in to do it. That vacation became for me the vacation we took because the baby wasn't born — and that even though I was pregnant again by then. (I lost that pregnancy to miscarriage, and as of the time I am writing this, I have not been able to become pregnant again.)

As time has passed, I do not have any regrets about the decision Daniel and I made not to bear a child with Down syndrome. Life — and in particular raising the children we already have — is challenging enough. I believe that my relationship with Daniel was changed by what we went through together. We weathered a crisis together. The intensity with which Daniel stayed close to me and supported me made me understand in new ways how much he loves me, and how much I love him. It is a wonderful thing to feel so well loved. We also learned how much our family and close friends love us. After we told them our bad news, some of them called every day just to let us know that they were thinking of us during that terrible time.

I will never think about abortion in the uncomplicated terms I did before my abortion. I have different feelings now about the question of when life begins, and at the same time I am more certain than ever of the importance of being able to choose whether or not to bear a child. Knowing what I now know about the type of abortion I had (in which the fetus has to be cut apart to be removed through the small cervical opening), which saved me the additional agony of going through labor, I understand why only a few doctors are able to perform the procedure, and I am grateful for the compassion and strength of every doctor who does, including the kind and gentle doctor who cared for me.

Those are the good things we took from the experience, and they are good things indeed. On the other hand, the pain of what we went through changed me and will always be part of me. I will always think about the baby we might have had. I will save the ultrasound picture of Bump in an album with the pictures of our other children.

6 ❧

The New Assisted Reproductive Technologies and Pregnancy Loss

Remarkable advances in the diagnosis and treatment of infertility have taken place during the past decade. At the present time the majority of couples who are diagnosed as having a fertility problem are candidates for some type of treatment. A fortunate few experience rapid success in becoming pregnant once treated, but more often the evaluation and treatment of infertility turn into an emotionally stressful, physically uncomfortable, time-consuming, costly, and demoralizing ordeal. It is not unusual for couples to spend years trying one treatment after another.

When a couple who identify themselves as having an infertility problem seek medical help, the first step is to diagnose the source of the difficulty. Testing will indicate if there is a male factor — that is, if the man's sperm are abnormal in number, morphology, or motility, or in their ability to penetrate an egg — or a female factor — if the woman does not ovulate, if her fallopian tubes are blocked, if she is not producing adequate levels of hormones, if her eggs are not fertilizable, or if she is producing antibodies to her partner's sperm. Sometimes testing indicates that both male and female factors are present. The diagnostic process should include examination of sperm and charting of basal body temperature to determine ovulation. Numerous other clinical examinations and tests are available and may be selectively ordered as indicated in each case. Once the evaluation has been completed and an understanding of the problem has been reached, a decision is made as to whether treatment is likely to be successful. If there is a range of treatments that may prove helpful, it is customary to begin with the simplest and least invasive procedure.

At the present time assisted reproductive technology is still in its infancy and should be considered an experimental procedure. There is no uniform standard that physicians can use to decide which assisted reproductive technologies (or ART) procedure to try with a particular couple, nor is there a standard way in which specific procedures are carried out. What this means is that before choosing an infertility specialist or center, you should ask for information on how patients are selected, what procedures are used, and what the "take-home baby" rates are.

A couple who have reached the point of trying to become pregnant through ART usually have already tried other interventions that have failed. Assisted reproductive technologies are a variety of techniques at the forefront of the field of infertility, designed to help couples with infertility secondary to tubal damage, endometriosis, male factor problems, immunologic difficulties, and cervical mucus disorders, as well as couples with unexplained infertility. All ART procedures are designed to bypass structural abnormalities in the female reproductive tract and to facilitate fertilization and implantation by removing these processes from the human body and placing them in the laboratory, where they can be controlled and modified. The most commonly used ART procedures are summarized below.

IVF (In Vitro Fertilization)
In this procedure, hormone treatment is first used to hyperstimulate the ovaries, or if this is contraindicated, the follicles are allowed to develop without intervention in a natural cycle. Laparoscopic surgery is then used to harvest the mature eggs from the ovary. In the laboratory the harvested eggs are exposed to sperm; fertilization takes place in a laboratory dish. After a few cell divisions, the fertilized eggs are placed in the woman's uterus through the cervix.

GIFT (Gamete Intrafallopian Transfer)
The initial harvesting process for this procedure is the same as that used in IVF. However, in GIFT the eggs and sperm are simultaneously placed in the fallopian tube, where fertilization can subsequently take place. This is a one-step surgical procedure.

ZIFT (Zygote Intrafallopian Transfer)
The procedures for ovarian hyperstimulation, harvesting, and fertilization used in this technique are the same as those used in IVF. In ZIFT, however, the undivided, fertilized eggs are placed in the fallopian tube, rather than in the uterus.

TET (Transuterine Embryo Transfer)
The first stages of this process are the same as those utilized in IVF and ZIFT, but after fertilization, cell division is allowed to continue, and an early embryo is placed in the fallopian tube.

Normally, the conception of a child is an invisible process; either it happens and you're pregnant, or it doesn't and you aren't. All this changes with ART, where each step of the process can be observed and thus determined to be successful or unsuccessful. The administration of hormones by injection or by ingestion allows for specific timing of ovulation; ultrasound lets your doctor track the number of follicles that are developing as well as their maturation. Together these procedures tell him or her if, when, and how many eggs will reach maturity. The surgical harvesting of eggs lets him or her know if retrieval has been successful and whether the eggs are of good quality. Similarly, when fertilization is done in the laboratory, the physician is able to determine whether or not this step has been successful. Finally, the β subunit HCG pregnancy test can tell doctor and patient whether pregnancy has occurred even before a period is missed.

Helpful and rewarding though it may be for many people, this unprecedented look into the process whereby pregnancy occurs also allows for more and earlier opportunities to experience loss and disappointment. Alice, forty-two, found that "everything in our life is tentatively arranged around a possible date for IVF or ZIFT. I am constantly vague about commitments during that ten-day to two-week span. If my results are good, I am elated but pressed to rearrange my calendar, stressed to keep our lives looking as normal as possible while arranging and waiting for the momentous, all-important surgical rendezvous. So much is riding on this date, so much reorganizing of priorities, so much hope for success. When a cycle is canceled, I feel devastated, morose, and exasperated. Many times I have sat in the waiting room, relegated from ZIFT to an IUI (intrauterine insemination). I felt left out and sad as I saw the other women being ushered in for egg retrievals. I couldn't help but think how well they responded, producing many eggs. I know that what I have is better than not ovulating at all, but it is painful for me."

It is impossible to go through an ART procedure without getting your hopes up, even if you know that the likelihood of success is not great. Fantasies about your future child may be present from very early on, as may feelings of attachment. Because it is possible to mourn the loss of a "hoped-for child," disappointment or grief may be experienced when any step in the ART process is not successful. Jane, forty years old, who had been in an IVF program for fourteen months, was candid about her despair and disappointment: "I had every reason to think I was pregnant. After so many failures and canceled cycles this year, I was happy to have a good natural cycle. It appeared from my temperature chart that my period was a week or more overdue. My hopes began to build with each passing day. I had a warm, visceral feeling of peace — maybe even joy (an emotion I don't think I've felt in almost two years). Try as I might, I could not help myself from bonding to the little being I hoped was there. I tried to suppress lovely visions of my new baby, but they came flooding through my imagination. 'All will be right with my world if you are there,' I said. Oh, the relief of it — the pure lovely luxury of being freed from this isolated heartsick state. In itself that was a reward. But to think I might have my baby, too! 'To finally see you in my life and hold you in my arms,' I mused. I wanted to leave this saddest of states so desperately that I let myself bask in the longed-for joy that I hoped would be mine.

"But no — the black reality came once again . . . my period. The vise of panic and despair closed itself upon my heart. A rush to the bathroom inevitably ended with a gasp of disbelief and uncontrollable sobs. Later the sadness and resignation gave way to bitterness, self-loathing, frustration, and anger. It will be a black night followed by several gray days as I regather my strength and resolve to resume another cycle.

"I feel the child I lost slipping further and further from me as each failed cycle lowers my statistical chances of ever being pregnant again. I weep again for my lost baby. The old yearning to hold it, nurse it, cuddle it, haunts me. All the things I have done to strengthen and nurture myself back to good health seem to have failed me. I know I will recuperate and move on. It is difficult, however, to live on these two levels — to try to function in the world while feeling so vulnerable, fragile, and sad."

As with any type of pregnancy loss, the emotional investment and the process of attachment may be quite different for each partner, and as is always the case, the potential for feeling emotionally isolated, misunderstood, and uncared-for is great. Since many couples keep their attempts at ART conception private, they cannot turn to family or friends for support when a loss occurs. This can place an enormous burden on the marriage: not only must partners try to understand those parts of each other's experience that are not shared, but they must do so at a time when their own resources are low. They may have difficulty comforting each other or need more than the other can give. Ann was grateful that her husband, Tom, was supportive. "All he can do to comfort me is to put his arms around me and stroke my head. He is anguished, too. 'I wish I could take away your pain,' he says in a desperate voice. If only he could."

All ART procedures have a rather low success rate: 15 percent per cycle at best. With repeated attempts, the likelihood of pregnancy is 15 percent per cycle for the first six cycles for couples under forty; after six cycles, the predicted pregnancy rate per cycle decreases. In couples over age forty, the likelihood that ART will be successful decreases after four cycles.

It is important to keep in mind that the pregnancy rate given in these statistics refers to the number of positive pregnancy tests, not to the number of live births. A positive pregnancy test is not a guarantee of success because the miscarriage rate is high with all ART procedures. In fact, couples may encounter failure anywhere along the way. They may have a poor response to the hormones used to regulate the cycle; no eggs at all or only a few mature ones may be produced; the harvesting process may be unsuccessful; the eggs, once harvested, may fail to fertilize; the fertilized eggs may fail to implant; and what appears to be a successful pregnancy can miscarry.

It is not unusual for couples to feel hopeful at the beginning of an ART cycle, increasingly anxious as they wait to find out if the procedure has been successful, and disappointed or even depressed if pregnancy is not achieved. Because ART procedures are extremely stressful, many centers require a psychological evaluation before accepting people into their program. However, even those deemed "psychologically capable" of coping may find it very difficult to deal with multiple attempts and repeated failures. To further complicate matters, some people are negatively affected by the hormone-treatment component of ART, and for all but the extremely wealthy or well insured, the financial cost of ART, which may run as high as $5,000 to $8,000 a cycle, is yet another stress. Some couples find the cumulative toll so incapacitating that they decide to stop trying. At the other end of the spectrum are couples who are unable to give up trying even though the likelihood of success appears to be low.

When, after an enormous investment of time, money, and emotional energy, a couple learn that they have had a positive pregnancy test, the last thing they want to think about is the fact that the miscarriage rate with all ART procedures is quite high. Unfortunately, since that is the case, all too frequently a couple's relief at learning that they are pregnant is followed by the disappointment of discovering that the pregnancy is not viable. In order to understand the full impact of losing an ART pregnancy, you have to understand what it is like to be infertile. An infertile couple have had to contend with the shame and disappointment they feel at not being able to become pregnant easily and on their own, as others do. In all likelihood they also have had to cope with an assault to their self-esteem, resulting in their feeling inadequate, undesirable, unattractive, and somewhat depressed. Furthermore, the many failures they may have accumulated on the road to ART have probably left them feeling fragile and all too familiar with grief, deprivation, and loss. Couples who lose an ART pregnancy often find that in addition to evoking grief for the child they have lost, the experience of miscarrying also reawakens memories of all the losses and disappointments they have suffered since first learning that they were infertile.

Liz miscarried a much-desired IVF pregnancy in her sixth week. "When I lost my baby, I entered a black hole of depression unlike anything I had ever known. I left the hospital a broken woman: I am totally broken in mind and body. My leaden feet carry me to the soothing solace of my darkened room and my safe, soft bed. My husband gives me a sleeping pill. I weep and plead for a deep sleep that will carry me far from the fields of my grief. I feel empty and lifeless, as if my life were a glass of water being poured out onto the floor. How can I live through these next few hours and days — my sadness is so utterly profound. I feel excoriated. I have nothing left. The trauma of loosing our long-yearned-for baby after all the infertility treatments has vanquished me. I am washed away as the leaves are washed down the storm drains by the heavy rain."

Many couples feel that both their individual and their joint reserves have been depleted by the infertility experience and that their ability to deal with additional problems has been impaired. They may also find that they feel angry and depressed and that these feelings interfere with their ability to be close, or, worse still, that they blame each other for their difficulties. If the cumulative strain is more than a couple can manage by themselves, they need to consider whether they can withstand the stress of continued infertility treatment, or whether they need to take a break or even stop entirely. Individual and/or couples counseling can be of help, as can infertility support groups.

ART is the last opportunity that many infertile couples have for producing their own biological child. While its use has resulted in the birth of many children to couples who would not otherwise have been able to have them, it is not always successful. Some couples endure many failed attempts before a viable pregnancy is achieved, while others, despite repeated tries, either do not become pregnant or fail to carry the pregnancy to term. The loss of an ART pregnancy is particularly devastating because it occurs after great effort and expense; because the couple may already be feeling beleaguered by what they have been through; and because for some this loss is the end of the road, and there is nothing more that they can do or try.

For a detailed description of the physical and emotional consequences of early pregnancy loss, see chapter 3.

One Woman's Story

I am now looking back over seven years. During much of this time I went through a series of infertility treatments ranging from hormones (Clomid and Pergonal) to a surgical procedure (GIFT). Along the way, I experienced many losses and one exhilarating win. I feel like a veteran who has retired from the war. It is hard to go back now to revisit what happened, but I want to tell my story. Although some of the details have gotten cloudy over time, the bottom line is pretty clear.

My husband and I had been together for ten years when we finally decided to get married. I was thirty-eight years old and relatively successful in my career as a landscape architect. He was thirty-seven and doing well in a real estate firm. One of the major reasons we were married was that we decided we wanted to have children. I immediately stopped smoking my ten cigarettes a day and began exercising more regularly to get my body in shape for the inevitable. Six months later a pregnancy test was positive. However, by the fifth week I was spotting. A later blood test confirmed that I no longer had a viable pregnancy.

My husband and I were confused and disappointed. We felt some rumblings of anxiety about whether this was "normal" or not. On the recommendation of a close friend, I went to see her fertility specialist just to confirm that there was nothing really wrong. We were on the fast track and needed to make this happen, much the way we were leading the rest of our lives.

Visits to the fertility specialist started out, and continued to be, anxiety-laden. It seemed as though the doctor saw me for a very short time when I was in his office and was reluctant to answer all my questions. I felt uninformed about what was happening, and I was unable to give my husband answers to the questions he asked me when I returned from each visit.

The doctor put both of us through a battery of tests that he assured us were standard. The results of a laparoscopy showed that I had a "stage I" endometriosis, which if treated would delay the possibility of my becoming pregnant. Based on the doctor's recommendation, we opted to put off the endometriosis treatment. The other tests did not show that either my husband or I had any clear abnormality or problem. My basal temperature charts showed that my ovulation was regular, though not as regular as it should have been. The upshot was that the doctor put me on the hormone Clomid.

About three months later I had a positive pregnancy test; we were off and running again.

Around the seventh week, while I was at work, I began to spot. This time I went home and went to bed and cried. My husband was deeply upset by the news; he felt I hadn't been taking it easy enough during my pregnancy. I received little sympathy and felt very alone. I dreaded the possibility that something might be really wrong. How could this be happening to me? Wasn't I healthy, strong, and always able to do what I wanted to if I was determined enough? When I went to the doctor's office a few days later, I miscarried right there. The lab analysis showed no particular abnormality — just a "blighted" ovum, as they call a pregnancy that wasn't meant to work.

The good news was that my body responded well to the Clomid, and I seemed to be able to get pregnant fairly easily. The bad news was that they didn't really know why I was miscarrying. After this, the doctor ordered chromosomal testing, which showed that I did have an abnormality that could cause Down syndrome and other disabilities as well as miscarriages. I didn't really mind hearing this news — at least someone had finally found something. It was scary, but a chromosomal abnormality could be tested for.

My memory becomes blurry here. I had another one or two miscarriages while on Clomid. Then I decided to change doctors. I was feeling a need for more individual attention. On the recommendation of another friend, who had just succeeded in having her first child after much difficulty, I went to see her doctor. He gave me new hope and a feeling that we would succeed together if we worked at it methodically. He took me off Clomid and let me return to my natural cycle.

This doctor determined that my problem could be what is called luteal phase deficiency, which is essentially a hormone deficiency after ovulation. He finally put me on a program of Pergonal, with progesterone supplements during the last half of my cycle. This program was problematic for me in several ways: it was very expensive, though luckily I had insurance that paid for most of it; it was somewhat painful, with many shots in the buttocks; and it was difficult logistically. Since neither my husband nor I was willing to administer the injections, I went to my doctor's office or to the hospital to get shots about fifteen days a month. In addition, I had to go to my doctor's office every couple of days to have blood tests and ultrasound examinations to monitor how the follicles were developing.

Scheduling all of this with a full-time job was very hard. I told only one woman at work about my infertility problems and treatments; she was going through the same thing herself. I was reluctant to tell anybody else, particularly my boss, since I was afraid of how it would affect my job prospects within the office. I had reached a senior position and didn't want to jeopardize it. The financial, emotional, and time commitment that this treatment required consumed my life.

After a few months on Pergonal, I had a positive pregnancy test. My husband and I were veterans now and knew not to get too excited. We just went about our daily business trying not to have many expectations. We didn't even talk to each other much about it.

When I got past the first twelve weeks, I got more excited and hopeful. When the nurse called to say that the amniocentesis results were okay, I couldn't believe it. I still cry today thinking how relieved and happy I was. I was five months pregnant, and we could finally tell people.

After that I relaxed and felt quite confident that everything was going to be all right. My husband never really stopped worrying. I don't think we had intercourse for the rest of the pregnancy since he was afraid of causing another miscarriage. When our son was finally born after forty-eight hours of labor, we felt he was truly a miracle child wrought by our doctor and high-tech medicine.

I turned forty-three one month after our son was born. It was a year and a half later before I even considered trying for another child. We were more than blessed with one, but maybe we might get lucky. It was difficult to face trying to get pregnant again since I knew so well what was involved. But I also felt a real urgency to move quickly due to my age. I was now forty-four. When I went back to see my doctor, he was quite guarded about our chances of success. I had crossed the line as far as age; forty-four was a lot different from forty-one or even forty-two.

Since Pergonal had worked in the past, the doctor put me on it again. What had been difficult before became almost impossible now. With a baby, a part-time job (twenty hours per week), and a husband who was struggling to set up his own business, I was overloaded. After three or four months on Pergonal, I didn't get pregnant. My doctor kept increasing the dose, but it didn't work. Then he told us that our only options were to quit or to go on to the next level of medical intervention, GIFT. He explained that the likelihood of success for me was 5 percent at best. He told us about what it would entail, including surgery. It all sounded very high-tech. On the one hand, I was excited by the possibilities; on the other hand, I wondered where this would end, this ever-expanding world of medical intervention. I wondered when the decision would be taken away from me — or would doctors be offering me possibilities until I was sixty-five?

How could I say no? We decided to go for it. All the monitoring, testing, and injections for the Pergonal program seemed to be doubled for GIFT. I lived at the doctor's office. I finally learned to give myself Lupron injections in the leg, and I also found a nurse who came to my house to give me the other injections I needed. The surgery that followed was not hard, but I was very uncomfortable and sore afterward. The surgeon reported that he was pleased to have found and implanted four healthy eggs. To everyone's great surprise, I got pregnant. I was the oldest woman in the clinic (and perhaps in the state) who had become pregnant using GIFT. My husband and I were incredulous and exhilarated. How had we been this lucky? We started to feel invincible. Everyone congratulated us. We went away on a trip out West, where I was very careful not to do anything like horseback riding or rafting. Another woman with us on the trip was also newly pregnant, so we did things together and talked a lot about having our second children.

The day we got home from the trip, I started bleeding. This was one of the worst moments. Soon after that, I went to see the obstetrician who had performed most of my D and C's. He was very loving and caring, as always. After the D and C, I felt very alone. I felt that something had happened maybe for the last time.

I did not feel the same after that. The old belief that we could somehow make it work was no longer there. I felt that my age was a problem and that the chances of our having a healthy baby were getting a lot slimmer. Perhaps it wasn't worth all the time, money, discomfort, and heartache.

Three or four months later, I found myself in a hospital emergency room, bleeding profusely. It turned out I was having a miscarriage without having known I was pregnant. This was actually not all bad news: I had gotten pregnant on my own, with no help from drugs or doctors. I had one more miscarriage after that, but nothing else has happened in the last year and a half. We have continued trying to get pregnant again on our own, but we have not really tried very hard. We are now considering adoption. My husband wants to give medical intervention one last chance, but I don't. I feel it is too risky for me at forty-seven. I'm not willing to go through the time, effort, and heartache it would take; I want to enjoy my son, my husband, and my life.

One last thought I want to share is that I don't think I grieved enough after each loss. I was so busy being a trooper, being strong and moving on, that I don't feel I cleared the air at each juncture. I tended to get numb, which is only apparent to me now. Eight miscarriages add up to a lot of loss.

7 🦋

Multiple Losses — When
It Happens Again

When you lost your first pregnancy everyone told you not to
worry — it happens to a lot of people. "Remember you are young
and healthy and have lots of time to have babies," they all said. And
you believed them, or at least you tried to.

It is hard to say when you began to believe that maybe they were
wrong. If you have not been able to become pregnant again, or if
you have and have lost these pregnancies too — chances are you are
not as hopeful as you once were. You ask yourself if you really want
to keep trying and when is the time to stop.

Other women seem to have babies so easily; why not you? Light-
ning is not supposed to strike twice in the same place, and certainly
not three times — or four times. Why is this happening to you? you
ask. You've suffered enough; you've paid your dues; you want a
baby more than anything else in the world. It just isn't fair.

After a while you feel convinced that there is something wrong
with you, that you will never have the child you want. You feel
damaged and incomplete. Sometimes you feel so frustrated you
could scream; some days you cannot shake your feelings of despair.
You blame yourself; you blame the world. You hate yourself for
envying other women and because having a baby is so important to
you. You can't help noticing that your obsession with having a baby
is taking a toll on you, on your family, and perhaps even on your
friendships. You want to go on with life — to have all of this behind
you — but there doesn't seem to be an end in sight.

The loss of a pregnancy is always painful, no matter if you have lost two pregnancies or ten. Consciously you may try not to be too hopeful, so as to protect yourself from disappointment if something does go wrong. Nevertheless, you can't help but feel disappointed if your pregnancy ends.

Most couples report that they have experienced increasing difficulty coping with each succeeding loss. Not only does one experience grief and mourning anew every time; eventually one starts to question whether something is seriously wrong and whether it will ever be possible to produce a child. In order that feelings of despair, hopelessness, frustration, jealousy, anger, and worthlessness not dominate one's life it is necessary to mourn each loss completely. Unfortunately, this becomes harder and harder to do, because as the blows accumulate, it is harder to put them behind you and your resources for doing so work less well. Some couples have found that their ability to recover disappeared completely at some point, and that although the acute pain diminished, they were left with persistent and unshakable feelings of depression. This was described variously as feeling that life had become "'dead," that it was hard to enjoy things, and difficult to feel excited by anything. Often despair looms so large that it takes over everything — every part of life is overshadowed by the pain.

Lisa and John sought counseling help after their third miscarriage because they felt that their attempts to deal with their difficulties on their own had not been successful. Lisa, a talented lawyer, had quit her job with a large law firm after her second miscarriage in the hopes that a less pressured existence would permit her to carry a pregnancy successfully. After three months of trying to conceive, she became pregnant. After two blissful months of pregnancy, she began to spot, and eventually miscarried. Both Lisa and John were devastated. They felt that they had done everything in their power to make this pregnancy successful. They felt helpless to do anything differently or better next time, and with this realization they felt totally at a loss. Lisa found that she was unable to think of anything else besides getting pregnant, being pregnant, and staying pregnant. She started to find it increasingly difficult to do anything outside the house, and for the first time in her life she even avoided friends. She felt acutely envious of several who had children, and found even telephone conversations with them agonizing. Worst of all, she was unable to tell anyone but John what was wrong. She had been raised to believe that she should keep her troubles to herself, lest other people think badly of her. Even though the isolation she was imposing on herself was unbearable, the thought that her friends or family would know how unsuccessful she was was even more painful. John, on the other hand, got to hear every detail of what she was feeling over and over again. Although he felt totally sympathetic and, in fact, shared her feelings, he found that a constant diet of grief was more than he could bear. He felt at a loss in remedying the situation, especially after they visited several new doctors, who found nothing conclusive. His decision to seek couples' counseling was reached when he recognized that not only was Lisa not getting over her grief, she was becoming increasingly depressed, and so was he.

Although they did not realize it at the time, both John and Lisa had been behaving in ways that were unproductive but that gave them some measure of control over what had happened to them: Lisa blamed herself instead of blaming fate, and John kept trying to make things better, despite the fact that there wasn't anything he or anyone else could do. These behavior patterns were not successful because they prevented the couple from coming to terms with the fact that sometimes in life things happen for no apparent reason and sometimes one is powerless to change them.

In therapy Lisa was able to separate her feelings about herself from her feelings about losing the pregnancies. She had originally experienced her miscarriages as tangible evidence of how inadequate she really was. Eventually, she came to recognize that although many unfortunate things had happened to her, this did not mean that she was bad or worthless. Once these feelings were resolved, she felt freer to let people know what she was going through, and to ask for their support. In addition, she began to enjoy life again and to recapture her optimism about the future.

Like Lisa, John discovered that he could not always be responsible for everything that happened. This realization allowed him to feel less helpless when he was unable to improve things. He was surprised to find that as he was more able to tolerate his own grief, his empathy for Lisa grew, thereby strengthening their relationship.

John and Lisa's situation is not unique. Although not everyone reacts the way they did, it is common to find that one's feelings about the actual loss are compounded by doubts, fears, or misgivings about oneself. These need to be dealt with so that needed energy is not diverted from the challenge at hand.

Why is it that, although most couples have no difficulty having a baby, some have so much? Doctors are not sure of how to answer this question, because although they know a great deal about why some couples have difficulty conceiving, and about why others lose their pregnancies, there is a lot that they don't know as yet.

If you have lost two or more pregnancies, or if you have been unable to become pregnant again after six months to a year of trying, your physician probably has suggested that you have a complete medical evaluation to determine the source of your difficulty. This evaluation may provide you with an explanation of why you have been having problems. There may be things that your physician can do to correct whatever may have been wrong. However, it may be that even a thorough medical evaluation will not succeed in turning up the source of your difficulties. As you know, it is often impossible to explain what caused a given miscarriage, stillbirth, or ectopic pregnancy. There is also much that is not known about why some couples experience multiple losses: repeated miscarriages, repeated stillbirths, or several ectopic pregnancies; or some combination of these. Similarly, more often than not, the reason why some women are unable to conceive, after having done so at least once, cannot be determined.

How long to keep trying is a highly individual decision. Many couples do finally succeed in having a child after numerous losses. Others have chosen to give up, some after one or two losses and others after many attempts. Still others have lost several pregnancies, then produced a child, later had more loses, and eventually produced more children.

Each couple must decide for themselves how much they can handle. Some things to think about in making this decision are: is there a known cause of our difficulties? If so, is there a specific treatment available, and what is the likelihood that it will be successful? If not, what is the likelihood that future attempts at pregnancy will be met with success? Also, can you cope with another pregnancy, and perhaps another disappointment? Alternatively, can you face giving up? Lastly, you need to think about alternatives such as adoption or childless living and decide if either of these is a choice you wish to make at the present time.

HABITUAL ABORTION

A concern commonly voiced by couples who have had a miscarriage is "What are the chances that our next pregnancy will be successful?" If you have not had more than one or two miscarriages, the answer to this question is quite encouraging. After one or two miscarriages, the statistical risk of having another is about the same as the risk of having one in the first place. This is because, in all likelihood, each was caused by random, unrelated events that have little likelihood of recurring.

A woman is said to be a "habitual aborter" if she has had three or more consecutive pregnancies that have terminated in miscarriage. Whether each of the miscarriages was caused by random factors or whether they were caused by recurrent, underlying difficulty must be assessed for each individual.

Studies of women who have had three consecutive miscarriages without a live birth have found that the chance that a fourth pregnancy will result in a live birth is somewhere between 20 percent and 80 percent. This range is too wide to be of help in predicting what the outcome of a particular woman's pregnancy will be. Moreover, all of these studies are based on a highly questionable underlying assumption: that all women who have had three miscarriages share a common difficulty, and therefore have the same odds of overcoming their problem. Unfortunately, none of these studies has investigated what the effect on the outcome of the pregnancy is of a specific problem, such as an incompetent cervix. Until specific problems are isolated and studied, the statistics will have little meaning. The risk of having another miscarriage for the woman who has cervical incompetence is, in fact, quite different from the risk for the woman whose husband is a carrier of a chromosomal abnormality and from that for the woman whose miscarriages were caused by unknown or random factors.

Most physicians recommend that a couple should be medically evaluated if they have had three consecutive miscarriages. However, many couples who have had two miscarriages are unwilling to attempt another pregnancy without knowing whether they may have a treatable problem, and so elect to begin an evaluation after the second miscarriage. It is likely that the physician will be responsive to a couple's preferences in this regard, so one should be sure to make one's wishes known.

In making his assessment your physician will be guided by his knowledge of your unique medical history, the course of each of your pregnancies, pathology reports on fetal tissue, if available, and what he finds when he examines you. A basic evaluation might include a hysterogram (dye is injected through the cervix in order to make the anatomy of the uterine cavity visible), and karyotyping (a study to determine whether either you or your spouse has a structural chromosomal abnormality). A more extensive evaluation might include thyroid function tests, a cervical culture for herpes virus and T-mycoplasma, measurement of serum progesterone, screening for systemic diseases known to predispose a woman to miscarry, and whatever other tests your physician believes may be fruitful.

REPEATED STILLBIRTH AND MULTIPLE LOSSES OF MIXED TYPE

Why some otherwise healthy women seem to be at an increased risk of experiencing repeated pregnancy loss is somewhat of a medical mystery, especially so since the majority of miscarriages and a significant number of stillbirths are caused by random, nonrecurrent factors. Stillbirth is often a result of either natural accidents of labor (such as prolapse of the umbilical cord, or placental abnormalities) or the injudicious conduct of labor or a traumatic delivery.

Less puzzling are those repeated pregnancy losses that occur in women who have either a chronic or recurrent illness or medical condition. There is a known correlation between certain medical problems and an increased rate of pregnancy loss. Among these are diabetes, kidney disease, systemic lupus erythematosis, severe hypertension, and toxemia. For example, the reported mortality rate for fetuses and newborns of diabetic mothers is 5 to 10 percent.

The chance that the fetus of a diabetic mother will be adversely affected is dependent to a considerable degree on how severe the illness is, how long the mother has had diabetes, and whether or nor she has preexisting kidney or blood-vessel damage as a result of her illness. Similarly, the risk of fetal loss associated with the other conditions listed depends to some extent on how severe the mother's illness is.

If you have had either a stillbirth or a combination of losses, it is critically important that you seek a thorough medical evaluation, preferably with a specialist in high-risk pregnancy. It is possible that you may have a diagnosable disorder, which can be treated, thereby increasing your chance of carrying a pregnancy successfully to term in the future.

Perhaps your problem is not that you don't know why you have lost pregnancies, but that you have to live with knowing that a disease or condition that you have was probably responsible for the reproductive difficulties you have experienced. If this is so, you may find that your ability to deal with both kinds of problems depends on how well you have accepted and accommodated to living with your illness. If you have had to make a major adjustment to living with a disease such as diabetes, you may have already come to terms with many of the issues one has to face when a pregnancy is lost. Having coped with this, you will probably have internal resources you can draw on.

If, on the other hand, you were minimally affected by your illness before you lost your pregnancy, you may find that it is particularly difficult to cope simultaneously with the grief that you feel at losing a pregnancy and the grief that you feel at recognizing that your illness has had a significant impact on your life. This may be the case for the woman with mild to moderate diabetes, for example.

ECTOPIC PREGNANCY: RECURRENCE AND SUBSEQUENT INFERTILITY

The incidence of persistent infertility and recurrent ectopic pregnancy following one ectopic pregnancy is significant. Studies show that 50 percent of women are unable to conceive after having had an ectopic pregnancy. This means that about half the women who have had one ectopic pregnancy will not be able to become pregnant again. Among those who are able to conceive, between 25 and 69 percent will have a subsequent normal intrauterine pregnancy; and between 7 and 12 percent will have another ectopic pregnancy. These statistics indicate that only about one third of the women who have had an ectopic pregnancy can expect to produce a living child.

What does this mean for you? Your chance of being successful may be better or worse than statistics predict, depending on whether or not the problem that caused the ectopic pregnancy involves both tubes or is confined to the affected tube alone; depending on the degree of damage caused by the ectopic pregnancy, on the surgical procedure your physician performed, and also depending on other factors that affect your fertility.

If during surgery your physician found that the affected tube was damaged beyond repair, and that your other tube was missing, malformed, or so damaged as to make the possibility of pregnancy unlikely, he will have informed you that your chances of conceiving without intervention are nonexistent. If, however, you still have one good tube on the opposite side, he will probably have removed the affected tube. (Leaving a damaged tube in place is considered unwise, because the likelihood that it will obstruct the passage of another ovum, thereby causing another ectopic pregnancy, is significant.)

A third possibility is that your affected tube was removed during surgery and that your remaining tube was found to be somewhat damaged. Depending on the extent of the damage, the likelihood that you will be able to conceive an intrauterine pregnancy without intervention may be either reasonably good or quite poor. In the latter instance reconstructive tubal surgery may be able to benefit you.

If the condition of your fallopian tube or tubes is not known, your physician will probably want to do a hysterosalpingogram. This involves inserting a special dye into the uterus through the cervix, and then monitoring by X ray its course through the fallopian tube(s) and into the abdominal cavity. By observing whether the dye moves freely through each tube, it is possible to determine whether the passageway is open or whether any obstruction is present. The results of this test will help your physician assess what your chance is of being able to naturally conceive an intrauterine pregnancy, as well as whether or not tubal reconstructive surgery is necessary and feasible.

At the present time, surgery to remove adhesions that obstruct the tubal passageway and surgery to reconstruct a damaged or malformed tube are the only treatments available to women who have obstructed or partially obstructed fallopian tubes. Whether or not these procedures are indicated, and what the chance is that they may be successful, should be assessed by your physician or, if he advises it, by a specialist whom he recommends. Tubal reconstruction is performed by only a small number of specialists; therefore, if it seems that surgical correction may be indicated, you will want to arrange to have a consultation with someone experienced with this procedure.

INFERTILITY

What few people realize is that fetal loss is a form of infertility. Although the term *infertility* is most often used to indicate an inability to conceive, it is also used to describe being unable to carry a pregnancy to term. Barbara Eck Menning, R.N., in her classic book *Infertility: A Guide for the Childless Couple*, defines infertility as the "inability to conceive a pregnancy after a year or more of regular sexual relations without contraception, *or the inability to carry pregnancies to a live birth.*"

Many couples who have experienced ectopic pregnancy, miscarriage, or stillbirth have a history of having had difficulty conceiving. In the case of ectopic pregnancy, the underlying cause of both infertility and fetal loss is often the same. On the other hand, the relationships among miscarriage, stillbirth, mixed and multiple losses, and infertility are not well understood.

The couple with a history of infertility is apt to feel a double sense of loss when a pregnancy fails, as it was probably long awaited and extremely precious. In addition, as there is a reasonable possibility that a future pregnancy will be hard to conceive, they may experience the lost pregnancy as the loss of their only opportunity to produce a child.

Infertility is painful and demoralizing. Years of trying to conceive, endless medical tests, basal body temperature charts, treatments, and "living by the menstrual cycle" all contribute to the stress that most infertile couples experience. So, too, do the feelings of anger, guilt, shame, sadness, self-doubt, and helplessness. Unfortunately, these painful feelings so familiar to the infertile couple are experienced anew when a pregnancy is lost. Moreover, the couple who has had to grapple with years of uncertainty about whether or not they would ever conceive is faced with a new set of obstacles: if they are able to conceive, will they be able to carry the pregnancy to term successfully? Or, as Lila and Joel put it, "Losing a pregnancy after five years of infertility was like being hit again after we had already been down for the third time. We had no resources left; we felt that all of the fight had been taken out of us; then along came another blow. We were aware of how difficult it was for us to get pregnant, and now it seems that getting pregnant is only half the battle."

An additional deprivation encountered by many couples who have conceived and lost a pregnancy after many years of being infertile is that of a support group. The infertile couple who loses a pregnancy may find that they receive little in the way of either sympathy or support from their infertile peers. When the wife was pregnant, they may have avoided or been avoided by those left behind. This self-protective distancing often continues, even though the pregnancy that began it has since failed.

Although, as a rule, infertile couples who are able to become pregnant are considered more fortunate than those who can't, it is not clear that this is, in fact, always the case. Not only is it extremely painful to lose a pregnancy, but paradoxically, the potential to become pregnant may stand in the way of successfully resolving one's feelings about infertility. The couple with no chance of becoming pregnant is forced to confront this very painful reality. When they have been able to do this, they are able to get on with their lives. The task for couples whose potential fertility remains unproven is more complicated. For them the prize is always just out of reach. It is hard to give up when, perhaps on the next try, one may be successful. So repeated attempts continue to be made, often delaying the successful resolution of their dilemma.

SECONDARY INFERTILITY

If you already have one or more children, but are unable to conceive or successfully carry a pregnancy, you are experiencing what physicians refer to as secondary infertility. Secondary infertility can result from any of the same causes as primary infertility. Secondary infertility is always frustrating and baffling. It may be hard to understand why, when everything worked the way it should the first time, you are encountering difficulty conceiving or carrying a pregnancy this time around.

Some couples who have lost a pregnancy find that although they did not have difficulty becoming pregnant the first time, they are not able to become pregnant again. More often than not, the reason is not immediately apparent, and it requires a careful infertility evaluation to diagnose the cause of the difficulty.

The couple who experiences secondary infertility after a pregnancy loss has a doubly heavy burden to bear. Not only do they suffer the loss of the child they were carrying, but in addition, they must contend with a second obstacle in the way of their desire to produce a child. Couples who are in this unfortunate position often find that their grief is quite prolonged. In part this is so because they are mourning not one but two very painful losses. Additionally, because they are unable to produce another child, this means of resolving their loss is not available to them.

Secondary infertility is similar to primary infertility, but in some important ways it is quite different from it. One of the central differences is one of self-definition. Couples who find that they have secondary infertility have not yet defined themselves as infertile. Likewise, since they already have a child or have been able to conceive, the outside world does not define them as infertile, either.

This can make for difficulty. Many couples have found that friends and relatives may either be unaware of their problem, or, if aware, may minimize it. After all, they were able to conceive or produce a child once, weren't they? What is frequently overlooked by outsiders is the couple's intense desire for another child and their pain at not being able to have one.

Because this often is not understood, the secondarily infertile couple often receives very little social support. Comments such as

"Don't worry, dear, you conceived once; of course, you'll be able to do it again" and advice to "get pregnant right away so your children won't be too far apart in age" reflect this attitude. So, too, do remarks intended as offerings of consolation, but often heard as insensitive and hurtful: for example, "Count your blessings; at least you have one" or "How much worse if this had happened to you the first time."

What others may not understand, and what secondarily infertile couples sometimes do not understand themselves, is that although already having a child may ease the pain somewhat, it does not necessarily diminish the longing to have more. Or, put another way, it is at once possible to feel fortunate that you have a child and quite miserable at not being able to have another.

III

The Experience of Those Close to You 🙘 🙘 🙘 🙘

8

Your Husband and Your Marriage

When a couple suffers a pregnancy loss a man is often faced with many burdens. He must help his wife get through the trauma, physically and emotionally. In addition, he must deal with doctors and tell the bad news to family and friends. Through all this, he must deal with his own emotions of shock, anger, and grief.

The man, too, has lost a child and his hopes and dreams for that child. He probably feels robbed and deeply saddened, yet he may find it difficult to express his feelings. His wife is probably too upset to comfort him, and he feels he must be strong for her and everyone else. Everyone turns to him, but he has no one to turn to. As a result, he may suppress his emotions and try to act as normal as possible. When asked how he is, he may say, "Fine," because he is too embarrassed to talk about his feelings, or fearful he will lose control.

It is likely that his wife is the main recipient of expressions of sympathy and concern. While he realizes that his wife has suffered even more than he has and is in need of support, he may still feel neglected or jealous of the attention she is getting. Alternatively, he may feel glad that no one is attending to his feelings, since he prefers to keep them invisible and under control.

During the actual loss many men feel afraid for their wives' health. Especially in the case of an ectopic pregnancy, there may be concern that the wife's life is in danger. If he is separated from his wife for any length of time, the man's fantasies may run wild: what if she doesn't make it? What if they can't stop the bleeding? What if she never comes out of the anesthesia?

Alternatively, he may have been with his wife during labor and delivery, possibly helping with the breathing techniques learned during childbirth classes. It is difficult enough for a man to watch his wife suffer the pains of childbirth when the result is a healthy baby. However, when the baby is dead, the suffering is even harder to bear.

The wife's stay in the hospital, no matter how long it was, is probably a time both would like to forget.

Bob, whose wife, Pat, stayed in the postpartum ward for three days following a stillbirth, describes his reaction to his wife's hospital stay: "The days when Pat was in the hospital were extremely hard on me. I spent as much time as I could at her bedside. I was the only one she wanted to see and I wanted to be with her. I hated watching the pain she was in and seeing her drugged. She was so upset, she cried almost constantly. I didn't know what to say to make her feel better. It seemed as if there were no words, so I held her a lot and told her how much I loved her and that we'd try again as soon as we could. I listened over and over again as she recounted the delivery and poured out her feelings. It nearly broke my heart to see her that way. At night I went home and cried myself to sleep."

If the pregnancy terminated in a stillbirth, hospital personnel probably consulted with the father about what arrangements to make for the baby's body and whether a funeral was desired. Some men make the decision themselves, preferring not to submit their wives to additional stress. Others consult with their wives to find out their preferences and to let them participate in the decision if they want to.

Regardless of the way it is handled, the question of making arrangements for the body of a stillborn child is probably one of the most unpleasant tasks a man has to face.

RETURNING HOME

The husband probably feels relieved and glad when his wife is discharged and able to return to the privacy of their home. At the same time, he may dread facing the enormity of their loss. He may have been able to keep up a front in the hospital, but at home he fears he will be overwhelmed by his emotions. He may also worry that his pain may be more than his devastated wife can bear.

In addition, he may be unprepared for the intensity of his wife's reaction to their loss. She is exhausted, in pain, depressed, irritable, and angry, unceasingly, it seems. She may cry a great deal and snap at him for no reason. It seems as if she is crying hysterically as he leaves for work in the morning; she is still in tears when he calls during the day to check on her; and the tears are still flowing when he comes home.

If she does not get over her grief, he may find that he craves some escape. It surprises him to find that he is tempted to get away, to work late, to take overnight business trips — anything to get a break. He knows he's a bastard for wanting to escape, but he can't stand it anymore. The fact that his wife can't escape, but he can, makes him feel all the more guilty for wanting to.

His efforts to cheer up his wife fail. He can't even get her to smile. He attempts to change the subject, but she keeps talking about the whole ordeal over and over again in explicit detail. He is sick of hearing about it and wishes she could put this behind her and go on with her life.

Her intense feelings of loss and sadness continue past the time he feels they should. Weeks or months have passed and she doesn't seem to be getting any better. He starts to wonder if there is something wrong with her — maybe she is neurotic; possibly she should see a psychiatrist or be hospitalized. During this period a man may be confused by his conflicting feelings toward his wife. On the one hand, he sympathizes with her pain and knows how important the baby was to her. On the other hand, he may be irritable with her and lack patience for her continuing grief.

DELAYED REACTION

A number of couples reported that the husband experienced a belated reaction to the pregnancy loss. As much as several months afterward, he may feel intense emotions not unlike what his wife felt immediately after the trauma. Initially he may have suppressed his own emotions in order to help his wife cope. As time passes and she begins to recover, he may find that his emotions surface and must be dealt with. All through the crisis, he had been able to carry on as usual at work and at home. Now he may be irritable, angry, jealous of couples with children, fearful of death, and depressed. He may never have experienced such strong emotions and may have difficulty expressing them. Because some weeks or months have passed since the loss, he may not even associate these feelings with the trauma.

Many men have been discouraged from showing their feelings. In this situation, however, it helps to let feelings emerge, to feel the pain, to cry. To recover fully, he too must pass through the various stages of mourning. (See chapter 1 for fuller discussion of grieving.)

THE MARITAL RELATIONSHIP

The loss of a pregnancy inevitably causes stress to each marital partner. Often the marital relationship is strained as well. However, despite the fact that the going may have been rough for a while, many couples have felt that sharing their grief over their lost pregnancy has brought them closer together. Sometimes we show a part of ourselves in times of crisis that we keep hidden at other times. Whatever the hidden aspect, whether it was an ability to cope, sensitivity, or optimism, there may be pleasure in discovering each other and in knowing each other more fully.

Some couples have found that they were strengthened as individuals and as a partnership by being able to comfort each other and by understanding what the other person was going through. To share feelings and to make it through together can lay the foundation for the development of a more trusting and intimate relationship. There is also satisfaction to be gained from feeling that one was faced with something hard, and that together, as a couple, the two of them were able to handle it.

One woman described the bond between herself and her husband following the loss of their pregnancy at eight months: "We went through it together, every step of the way: the pain, the hope, the anger, the feelings of isolation, and the decisions at each step. I couldn't imagine not having him to share it with. We cried together and got angry together. Our relationship grew stronger as he and I together faced all the babies and pregnant ladies in the grocery store."

Another woman, Sarah, spoke of the effect her stillbirth had on her relationship with her husband, John. "We became closer than ever. John was not ashamed to cry in my arms, nor I in his. The grief would not hit us at the same time during the months that followed, but we were always sensitive and supportive when it did hit. My husband was very upset, and during this time, for the first time ever, I saw him cry. I know he was very hurt. We both wanted the baby desperately. John still has a special spot on his jogging trail on the top of a mountain, where he stops to think about her."

Sarah's words reflect the thoughts of many women. Her husband's reaction to the loss helped her become aware of the depth of his love and devotion. Coming at a time of great vulnerability, this reassurance was especially welcome.

She took comfort in the fact that John grieved over the loss and she felt better knowing that he, too, was hurt and had yearned to have a child. She felt optimistic that they would be parents someday, either by giving birth or by adopting. Knowing that John wanted a family as much as she did helped Sarah cope with her grief and look toward the future.

PULLING APART

Pregnancy loss can strain even the best of relationships. Couples who have relatively stable and longstanding relationships may find themselves arguing, feeling misunderstood, resenting one another, or withdrawing completely.

If this is your experience, you may find this fracture in your relationship distressing. After all, you are in the middle of a crisis, and feeling close to your spouse is more important than ever. Friction between you only adds to your tremendous emotional burden. It is not uncommon to feel as if everything were going wrong all at once. First, you lost your baby, now you feel at times as if you are losing your husband, and maybe your mind. Try to remember that both of you are going through a crisis and, given the complex nature of what you have been through, there is no end of opportunities for communication to break down.

To understand why problems so frequently arise, it is important to realize that the psychological experience of losing a pregnancy is likely to be very different for each parent. Most women form an emotional attachment to their future child early in the pregnancy, while most men feel little or no attachment until late in the pregnancy, or form an attachment only after the child is born. This is because the woman experiences pregnancy more directly — she senses the early signs and symptoms and later feels the baby move inside her. Early on, a husband can experience the pregnancy only through his wife's words and observations. A woman who suffered two miscarriages commented: "A man doesn't sense the physical bonding a mother does. I don't think my husband related to the fetuses as babies — real persons. He did not have the physical pain, humiliation, or hormonal ups and downs that I did. He surely wasn't happy about these miscarriages, but he did not experience the losses as strongly or significantly as I did."

It follows, then, that because each parent has a different attachment, each will have a different response to the loss of a child early in pregnancy. The mother may mourn the loss as she would the loss of a beloved person. The father in all likelihood has not yet formed a strong attachment to the child, and therefore his grief will probably be less profound and of shorter duration.

"My husband was understanding but couldn't know what this did to my whole sense of myself," said Karen following her miscarriage. "After months of my moping and lack of interest, he wondered if I wasn't prolonging things and overreacting. I started resenting him for having escaped the full emotional burden of the loss. It was a difficult time for us. I think it is impossible for a man to understand miscarriage on anything but an intellectual level."

When partners do not understand that each of them has formed a different kind of attachment to their future child, they are likely to be confused and angered by their spouses' response to the loss. The husband may feel that his wife is overreacting and she may be furious with her husband for being less affected than she is by the loss.

Donna describes her experience: "In a moment of tenseness, when we were both exhausted, he finally confronted me with his feeling that by this time I should have had more perspective.

His insensitivity confirmed my estrangement from him. I also felt foolish at not having realized before that we were so different."

The duration of the pregnancy may partly determine how the husband reacts to the loss: the longer the pregnancy, the more attached he is likely to feel to the baby. In the case of ectopic pregnancy, the husband may not have known of the pregnancy before it was discovered. Even if he did know, his wife was probably no more than two months along. Similarly, when miscarriage occurs early in pregnancy, the husband has had little or no time to get used to the idea of having a baby or to become emotionally invested in the pregnancy. Carol, who miscarried at four and a half months, remarked: "I was totally disappointed in my husband at the time. As far as he was concerned, there really was no pregnancy. He could not experience the grief that I was going through. He was very sympathetic to my fears but not to my grief. I often said to him that I wished that I had broken an arm or a leg so that he could see my wound and understand."

The father is apt to be most affected when the loss occurs late in pregnancy or when a child is stillborn. As many months have passed, he, too, has experienced fantasies of the expected baby. Chances are he has put his hand on his wife's abdomen to feel the baby kick or has heard its heart beat. When his future child has become a reality to him, he is likely to mourn its loss in much the same way as his wife does.

RECOGNIZING THAT EACH PERSON MUST MOURN IN HIS OWN WAY AND IN HIS OWN TIME

When couples are able to share their feelings, they are better able to resolve their misunderstandings, especially when one partner is mistaken about the other's emotional state. Judy told us: "My husband was a bulwark of strength throughout everything. With my first miscarriage my husband was told by my mother to be strong for my sake. I found this out much later. This caused him to cover up his grief. I attributed his normalcy to lack of caring. Communication between us broke down almost entirely. It took months for him to admit that he was in pain just like me. We learned from our past experience and grieved together after our second miscarriage."

Patty reports a similar experience after her ectopic pregnancy. "He was more upset than I realized as he tried to hide his feelings. I felt bitter and angry at the world that I had lost a baby and then had to go through the discomfort of surgery, too. Not until several months after the ectopic pregnancy were my husband and I finally able to share our feelings. We cried together and then felt much better. I think each of us tried to put up a front for the other. My husband's grief was as deep as mine, but I didn't know it at first. There was a lot of tension during the several months when I felt he wasn't disturbed much at all. Since we finally had it out and I learned his feelings, everything has been fine."

Some women viewed their husbands' reactions to the loss as typical of their way of coping with crisis. Their husbands' style was to grieve for a short time, get over it quickly, and go on with life. These men often failed to understand that their wives needed more time than they did to get over the death.

"My husband's grief was equal to mine, but he resolved it sooner," Joyce said. "He cried a lot the first day but composed himself a lot more quickly than I did. He generally accepts things better than I do. He doesn't dwell on something. He prefers to accept and set things aside — to go on in a positive fashion. He thought my feelings should have been handled and let go sooner than they were. He viewed my grieving as unnecessary and counterproductive. He kept telling me it was in the past and I should go on with my life."

Another women, Sandy, said of her husband: "He was unhappy to lose the baby but felt there was no point in mourning what could not be changed. He was more upset for me than for himself. Ultimately, he was disturbed by the fact that I could not get over my grief. He felt badly for me, yet he simply did not understand me."

Hurt feelings and fears that your husband does not share your grief are not easy to cope with. Try to give your partner the benefit of the doubt. It is likely that he is suffering, too. Put yourself in his place and try to imagine how you would react. In addition, try not to assume anything. Before interpreting your spouse's behavior, ask him what it means. You may save yourself a lot of pain and grief.

Communicate your feelings to each other. What you're going

through is real and deserves to be shared. Sharing your feelings should help you to grow as individuals and as a couple.

"I tried to push my husband away at first," said Lynn. "I felt that losing him would be just punishment for someone like me who couldn't even perform a normal biological function. I finally realized that losing him would be worse than losing the baby. Our marriage has been loving, strong, and happy ever since."

Try to resist the temptation to withdraw from your spouse. You need one another now. If you notice that your partner is emotionally isolated, make a special effort to open lines of communication.

One woman commented: "Since we weren't able to talk, my husband took a position where he traveled a lot, and wasn't home very often. This led to more misunderstanding and almost to the breakup of our marriage. We couldn't help each other work through our loss, so we felt sad and alone."

Another said: "I couldn't talk to my husband about feelings that made sense to him. I cried a lot, sat and didn't talk for an hour at a time. It frustrated him. Neither of us knew how to cope."

SOURCES OF MARITAL TROUBLE

Many spouses experience difficulty understanding each other's feelings after a pregnancy loss. It is often difficult for the husband to comprehend the intensity of his wife's pain, since he did not share her physical experience of the pregnancy or her strong emotional attachment to it. Similarly, it may be difficult for the wife to appreciate her husband's pain. If he is not open about his feelings or if she is so depleted by her own physical and emotional anguish that she is unable to be aware of anything else, she may fail to recognize that he too is grieving.

Difficulties may also arise if a partner openly or secretly blames the other for doing or not doing something that may have affected the outcome of the pregnancy: for example, participating in an activity such as sports, work, or travel. Sometimes one partner may blame the other for having had ambivalent feelings early in the pregnancy, as in the following situation. "The pregnancy was not a loss to him. It didn't represent a baby as it did to me," said a woman who miscarried at almost four months. "I developed a great deal of resentment for what I felt was his lack of grief and never hesitated to say, 'Well, you never wanted that baby anyway.' "

One spouse may project his or her own ambivalence onto the other spouse and then feel angry with him or her for having those feelings. If you find you are blaming your spouse for causing the loss, stop and think. Maybe your need to blame comes from your own anger, guilt, or need to find a reason. Remember, it is very unusual for pregnancy loss to be caused by something anyone did. Similarly, if your partner blames you for causing the loss, help him or her see that it was no one's fault. It may be helpful for both partners to visit their doctor together to hear his explanation; any questions about possible causes can be resolved at that time.

It is not uncommon for one or both partners to fear that they will be abandoned by a disappointed or angry spouse. Some couples "act out" these fears by testing or provoking each other. In the following case, the wife acted on a mistaken assumption. After her second miscarriage, Miriam felt convinced that her husband of five years would surely want to leave her to marry a woman who could have children. She began to withdraw and to become increasingly unavailable to him to minimize the hurt she would feel when he actually left. Although he was patient at first, Carl eventually found himself increasingly irritated with Miriam's withdrawal. During a major confrontation between them, Carl told Miriam that he felt emotionally abandoned by her, and she was able to tell him of her fear that he would leave her. Had they been unable to talk about their fears, Miriam might have continued to behave in such a way as to bring about the reaction from Carl that she dreaded most.

Another difficulty sometimes encountered by couples who have lost a baby is that either partner, or sometimes both partners, may experience a short-lived or longer-lasting decrease in sexual desire. This may be the result of an underlying depression, or it may be related to anxiety, feelings of inadequacy, fear of conceiving another pregnancy, or pressure to conceive again. One or both partners may feel that sex has become a chore. "Sex wasn't fun anymore" is the way one woman expressed it. The anger, fear, or anxiety thus engendered may further compound already present problems.

Try not to panic about your sexual difficulties. Most likely, they are a reaction to stressful circumstances and will improve as time passes and as you and your partner begin to feel better.

Counseling should be considered if after several months have passed either or both of you continue to feel emotionally estranged, angry, depressed, uninterested in sex, or unable to function. The loss of your pregnancy may be the first crisis you have faced together, and you may need help in dealing with it. Counseling can help you define your problems and cope with them more effectively.

One Man's Story

My wife, Alaina, gave birth to our daughter by cesarean section; I was present at the delivery. I was as unprepared initially for the stillbirth as the doctors were. Our baby had four congenital heart defects, which were undetected during pregnancy (through no fault of our obstetrician) due to the fact that while the baby was in the womb, Alaina's body supplied the necessary biological functions to keep the baby alive, masking the heart deficiencies. During delivery, when she was subjected to stress and when Alaina's life-support systems were removed, our daughter was not able to survive on her own. The thought that maybe something could be wrong with our baby had occurred to Alaina and me but, like many parents-to-be, we had given it little serious thought.

Within the space of a few short hours we experienced the thrill and excitement of expecting an apparently perfect child, and then the blackest despair when we discovered that our baby had died.

When the doctors quietly told me that our baby was dead, it didn't matter to me that they were in tears or that the nurses were obviously deeply affected. Alaina and I felt alone, deserted by life. We didn't want to talk with anyone about what had happened, because we felt so alone and helpless. We found ourselves searching for answers, for solutions to the emotional turmoil we were experiencing. It was a very personal grief, which continued for days and weeks afterward.

Where could we turn for help? Friends? Our parents? Doctors, nurses?

Immediately after the doctors gave us the bad news, I phoned my father and Alaina's parents with the news. They would then tell others in our immediate families, as I was too upset to do so. Sometimes it is hard enough for a person to cope with his own emotions, much less those of others.

Alaina and I felt that it was important that an autopsy be performed, since we hoped to learn what had caused our baby to die and thus, if possible, to prevent such occurrences in the future. Our consent was required, and I had to sign a form giving the doctors permission. I felt almost as if I had received a physical blow as I signed my name to that piece of paper.

Immediately after our daughter's death Alaina and I wanted to be alone; we felt too emotionally drained to deal with others just then.

I remained with Alaina in the hospital for two days, in the same room, sleeping in a recliner chair the nurses had thoughtfully provided; they realized what Alaina and I were going through and were magnificent in their understanding and generous with their help. The maternity ward personnel were very aware of life and death and the impact of both on the parents. Alaina and I needed each other very much, and this time was quite important for us. Little was said, but the fact that we were together was a comfort. I ignored my job and outside responsibilities. I felt that my first responsibility was to Alaina; everything else was secondary. I stayed with her constantly, attending to her needs, simply being there to help if she needed me.

After the first heartbreaking hours passed, the relatives had been notified, the various official forms had been signed, and other details completed, I was in a state of physical and mental exhaustion. I had not slept more than three hours at a stretch in three days. Whenever I went home to rest after those initial days, I always returned as quickly as possible; I felt very uncomfortable when I was not with my wife.

When I was home, our son, Christopher, and I were together constantly. After telling him what had happened, I answered his questions about his baby sister and about why she wouldn't be coming home to her new room that he had helped us decorate. I was amazed at the wealth of understanding Christopher displayed; he was hurt, sad, and confused, but he always told me: "I love you, Daddy, and I won't go away." He wasn't very old at the time, just past three, but he grasped what had taken place and, with the innocence of the young, helped his daddy to cope with it. He has always been a special boy, and is even more so now.

I assumed much of the burden of worldly affairs. I had to make various arrangements, and I had to act as a buffer between Alaina and the world in general. There were many things that had to be dealt with, important issues that could not wait, that had to be faced. For instance, I had to decide who visited, the length of time visitors remained, and the emotional and physical impact these visits might have on Alaina.

Although people mean well, care for you, and want to help, visits can be tiring. We found that both of us were gladdened at the display of concern but at the same time exhausted by it. In general, we tried to keep visits short.

After three days Alaina was moved from the maternity section to the surgery recovery floor. Because she had had a cesarean section, the time she spent in the hospital was longer than for a normal delivery. The psychological implications of this move, we found, were enormous and difficult. Her removal from the ward concerned with new life and happiness to another dedicated to recovery from physical trauma caused us both pain; the last link between us and our baby had been severed.

We found that the nurses on the surgery ward didn't know what had happened to us. At least four nurses asked either Alaina or me how our new baby was doing. It became annoying the second, third, and fourth times I had to explain that our daughter had died.

Alaina was released from the hospital after nearly five days, and we finally found ourselves at home. Before she came home, I did whatever household chores were necessary and had everything ready for her return; it didn't seem right to have her come home to anything other than a clean house.

Just as we had started to recover, reality struck again; the baby's burial had to be arranged. Earlier, while we were still at the hospital, I had made arrangements with our local mortuary to transport the body to their facilities for cremation. One of the worst experiences I had was going to the mortuary to obtain our daughter's ashes. I held them in my hands; a small wrapped box of ashes was all that remained of our hopes and dreams.

When the plot and headstone were ready, my father kindly took the ashes to the cemetery, had them buried and the headstone installed. The ashes were interred with my grandfather and grandmother in our family plot in a quiet, tree-shaded cemetery in a small rural town where my father and his family grew up.

After this was done Alaina and I had to make the decision as to whether we wanted to have a funeral service or not. We did not have a service. We felt that our baby was too new to the world for others to feel as strongly about her as we did. We also felt that a funeral service would only compound the grief we already felt. Outside pressures (societal, family, religious, and so on) were strong, but I made it known to everyone who mattered that our mutual decision was not to have a formal service. Alaina and I would take care of it in our own way.

Soon after our arrival home, doctor bills, hospital bills, and other reminders began to arrive. These were a continual reminder of what had taken place. The past kept intruding into the present: this went on for months, especially when we began receiving advertisements for various new-parent and new-baby magazines.

Friends and family sometimes offered their opinions, thoughts, and suggestions about what we should be doing, both for the moment and in the future. The flow of comments and advice began about a week after we had lost the baby. The absolutely worst things that were said to us were "Well, it just wasn't meant to be." Or: "It's God's will." Or: "You and your wife are being tested." Or: "Forget about having children and just proceed as if nothing happened. Do what you want to do and forget about kids."

We listened politely, nodded our heads, and then ignored, or tried to ignore, what had been said. We knew we would decide what was right for us. However, after hearing the same "suggestions" over and over again for weeks, I found it increasingly difficult to remain silent. Once, I even blew up at an acquaintance who gave me the "You're being tested" line.

I myself was more than a little bitter about what had happened. If what happened to us was a "test," then it was a grotesque and cruel test that was totally unnecessary. I couldn't comprehend then, and I don't now, any reason for what happened to our baby and our family. We had done everything correctly, had not endangered the unborn child in any fashion, and had every reason to expect the delivery of a perfectly healthy and normal child. I am still upset that our child was taken from us; it was not fair. It was cruel. This reaction is, I feel, perfectly justified and normal; I have no guilt about feeling as I do, and I expect others to respect my feelings.

After I had been back at work for two weeks I found that I was dreading going to the office. In my business, I deal with the public; this meant that I had to explain two or three times a day that our baby had died. Some well-meaning person would ask how our new little one was getting along, and I then had to go over it all again.

Our depression and unease continued for months; at first, we felt down much of the time. As the days passed, however, our outlook gradually improved, and emotional lows occurred less frequently. Still, grief continued to strike periodically for weeks and months afterward. We weren't prepared for this, and it was rough.

Often I struggled with my emotions and my memories of all that had happened. I couldn't keep all of the emotional by-products bottled up inside; I am thankful to have some close friends with whom I was able to discuss what I was feeling. I found that it was good to be able to talk to someone outside the immediate family at times. Mostly, it was helpful to talk with Alaina. I found that sharing our feelings with each other brought us closer together than we had ever been. We had planned together for our child, prepared ourselves for the new addition, dealt with the pregnancy for nine months, attended the birth, and coped with the death together, Alaina and I.

And yet . . . our baby is gone.

9 🎋

Children, Family, and Friends

Besides your spouse, the other members of your immediate family affected by your pregnancy loss are your children. One dilemma of parenthood is introducing and handling the topic of death. What do you tell your child? How many details? How can it be described so that he or she understands and is not frightened? At what age are children aware of death? All of these same questions and concerns arise when a pregnancy is lost.

Since pregnancy loss and death are uncomfortable topics, there is a tendency to want to avoid them as much as possible. We convince ourselves that a grandparent's death can be explained by saying he went away on a long trip. We want to spare our children exposure to sadness and the trauma of a death in the family. After an early pregnancy loss, we tell ourselves that a young child couldn't know that anything unusual has happened, and that therefore we need not tell them what has gone on.

When we do not deal with death openly and sensitively, our children sense that this is a topic that can't be talked about. Although our intention is to protect them from a painful and uncomfortable issue, unfortunately we teach them that death is something to fear, something so bad that it can't even be discussed. Children will remain silent about the loss of a pregnancy if they think that the subject is taboo. Not knowing what actually happened, they may create fantasies that are often more frightening to them than the real tragedy. (Children frequently deal with the unknown by creating a fantasy to explain things.) Thus, wrapping the loss in silence and secrecy can lead to worse fears than the reality would.

Besides, such secrecy is usually unsuccessful, because children tend to be keenly aware of everything that goes on in the family: they sense sadness, tension, and subtle changes in their parents' behavior. They also have a way of overhearing conversations, of being awake when we are sure they are asleep, and of seeing and hearing more than we are willing to acknowledge. Moreover, most children are able to read the subtle cues (through body language, for instance) that indicate what your real feelings are, even if you try to hide them.

"When I came home from the hospital, my son would sit next to me and hold my hand," one mother said. "It was sweet and comforting. He didn't even know about the miscarriage, but he seemed to sense that something was wrong."

How your child will experience the loss of your pregnancy is determined by many factors: his age, his personality, his past experiences with death, his awareness of your pregnancy, what he witnessed of the loss, how you reacted to the loss, and how you responded to him during this time.

Initially, most children are puzzled and confused. They want to know what happened, why it happened and how. In answering these questions, it is important to remember that your child's understanding is limited by his current level of development. He may not be able to comprehend what you tell him about the death of a potential sibling, but the discussion of it with him will set a pattern of openness and sharing.

In preschool children, several factors may account for confusion or fear about death. The young child has difficulty grasping the finality of death, for one thing. Also, young children often think of themselves as the center of their own world and therefore responsible for everything that happens in it. Further, they have a strong belief in magic. If the child is angry with you, he or she may wish for you to disappear or die. After learning of an expected new child, he or she could feel threatened or jealous and wish the baby would disappear or die. Consequently, if the baby dies, the child may feel that his or her wish caused the baby's death. She or he needs to be assured that this was not so. It is important she or he knows that these wishes did not hurt either you or the baby. If the child believes that he or she caused the baby's death, he or she might come to feel that aggressive wishes could cause other tragedies and may become fearful of the power of his or her own thoughts.

The best way to avoid such fears is to supply your child, even if he or she is quite young, with a clear, simple explanation, appropriate to the child's age, that will give him or her a real way of understanding what happened. For example, one might tell a very young child: "The baby was born when it was too small to live, so we are not going to have a new baby." It is not necessary, or even desirable, to give children all the details. Tell them just enough to make the issue comprehensible, then let them take the lead in asking you what they want to know.

SUGGESTIONS FOR DEALING WITH YOUR CHILD

The following is a model for dealing with your child's thoughts and feelings about the loss. It is based on suggestions discussed by Carol Hardgrove and Louise Warrick in "How Shall We Tell the Children?"

Offer a simple, clear explanation in language and concepts understandable to a child of his or her age. For example, here is what one couple said about telling their four-year-old: "We told her that it was not a baby but a seed for a baby. Later, we told her not all seeds grow. She had this concept from growing a garden."

Use correct words, such as *death* and *died,* rather than euphemisms. Describing death as a long sleep, for instance, may bewilder children and even cause them to fear sleep. Such a comparison and other distortions of death should be avoided, for they may bring more problems in the long run.

Elicit your child's thoughts and feelings. This is best done by asking questions such as "Have you been thinking about the baby a lot?"

If your child does not ask questions spontaneously, take the initiative and seek his or her own explanations of how babies develop, how they are born, and what he thinks happened to the baby you were carrying. This gives you important cues as to what information, corrections, and explanations are needed.

Answer questions when you are asked. One useful way of dealing with them is first to ask your child the same question you have just been asked. For example, when your child asks you what happened to the baby, you can respond: "What do *you* think happened?" In this way, children can express their concepts and feelings while providing you feedback to help you deal with them.

If you use books to explain, you should be familiar with the content before introducing them to your child; then you can discuss the material with her or him. Simply handing the child a book and suggesting he or she read it indicates that you are uncomfortable with the subject and implies that birth and death cannot be spoken of. Several books are listed in the bibliography.

If your child is familiar with religious beliefs, death can be discussed in a religious way, such as that the soul went to heaven or the baby is an angel now. It is best to avoid an expression such as "God took the baby" lest the child become afraid of being taken next.

Continue to raise the matter of the baby's death for months afterward. Also make it easy for your child to raise questions or talk about what happened. Parents should realize that the loss of a pregnancy, though once explained, may dwell in children's thoughts and come up again. Children usually need time to ponder, to understand. Questions will arise weeks or months later, either because something new has happened in their world or because they have reached a new developmental level that makes certain new concepts possible.

Convey to children that there is nothing that cannot be talked about, no question that cannot be asked. However, parents do not need to pretend that they have all of the answers. It is all right to say, "I don't know why that happened."

Respect children's defenses. They do not need, nor will they profit from, an overdose of reality. It is not necessary or advisable for children to accept and assimilate everything all at once. Give them time.

Be expressive of your own feelings of sadness and don't hide them from your child. This will allow him or her to express feelings of sadness without being in a position of needing to protect you from his or her feelings.

CHILDREN'S REACTIONS

Each child reacts uniquely to his mother's losing a baby. Even children who have been carefully prepared often behave in unexpected ways. Since this is a new experience for you and your child, there is a large element of uncertainty that makes it difficult to anticipate exactly what the effect will be on him.

In understanding your child's reaction, you should keep in mind that you may not immediately comprehend how he or she experienced the loss or what he or she believes happened. Very young children may be unable to verbalize their thoughts about it. If they feel guilty or responsible, if they feel that somehow they killed the baby or that you did, or if they feel disappointed or deprived, their reactions are apt to reflect this.

"Our four-year-old was disappointed and frustrated when we told her," one mother said. "She asked, 'Is it because you didn't take care of it?' 'No,' I replied, 'I did everything I could. It just wasn't the right seed.' She said angrily, 'Well you should have gotten a book that told you the right way to take care of it.' "

In addition, your child's reactions will be less baffling to you if you remember that children grieve differently from adults. Some psychiatrists think that children are incapable of true mourning until adolescence. Before this time, they do not really have the ability to understand death or to cope with it by internalizing the loss. If you don't understand this, your child's apparent lack of concern or newly acquired behavioral problems may be confusing. Children often express feelings of grief in their actions rather than in words. Some children may appear whiny and difficult, others may be aggressive or destructive; still others may be angry, withdrawn, or clinging. Be on the lookout for unusual behavior, which may be an indication that your child is struggling with painful feelings or frightening or disturbing thoughts or fantasies.

A mother who miscarried said: "Our daughter seemed fine all along and then one day she tried to push the fish tank over. I was shocked, as she was always so perfectly behaved. After much discussion, she was able to tell me that she thought that if the baby died inside of me, I would die, too. I assured her that this was not so. She wanted to know how the baby would get out, or if it would just stay inside me. I explained fully and factually. After that, she had no more fears or behavior problems and was fine."

Following is a small sample of the ways in which some children have reacted to the death of a potential sister or brother.

"Our four-year-old's grief was not as obvious as ours after the stillbirth. He cried when we told him of her death. I noticed that his finger paintings became very dark, colorless, and shapeless for a couple of months. He still talks about her and wishes that she was here to play with him."

"Our two-year-old was angry, sad, and disappointed. She reflected our sadness. A few months later our three-year-old suddenly became clingy."

A third mother remarked: "After my ectopic, my two-and-a-half-year-old son was very upset about my being in the hospital and away from him. It took him a number of months to accept having a babysitter after that."

It is important for parents to read behavioral signs that indicate distress. If troubling behavior is present, you should try to determine what may be bothering your child. If the child is verbal, ask him or her what he is worried about, or suggest areas of concern that you think might be disturbing him. If the child can't express himself verbally, situation role-playing may be useful. Similarly, parents can use dolls or storytelling to help their children talk about events that occurred in the life of the doll or fictional character, which mirror events in the child's own life. For example, you could start a game by saying, "When mother doll went to the hospital . . ."

Some parents have found that the family physician or the child's pediatrician may be willing either to offer advice on how to deal with the child's concerns or to deal directly with the child. If this latter situation occurs, it is critical that you be present when the doctor speaks with your child.

Occasionally, a child may have a significantly disturbed reaction to losing a potential sibling. Any intense reaction that does not seem to diminish spontaneously over time is a cause for concern and should be discussed with your pediatrician. He or she may be able to offer you valuable suggestions for helping your child. He will also be able to assess whether counseling may be useful in helping your child deal with his feelings.

ANTICIPATING THE CHILD'S NEEDS

The parent who recognizes that his child may be affected when a potential sibling is lost is in a position to anticipate his very special needs during this difficult time. First, you should be aware that the issue of death is frightening to almost all children. Like adults, they may feel an increased sense of personal vulnerability when someone close to them dies. "After my stillbirth," Alice said, "my three-and-a-half-year-old daughter asked me endless questions about dying. She became fearful of death since she knew it would mean that she'd never see us again."

One way to diminish your child's feelings of vulnerability is to point out that he or she is not in danger. A simple statement such as "The baby was very small and not strong enough to live yet; not like you, you're a big, strong, and healthy child" should help him or her to feel safer. Physical closeness with children is another way of telling them that they are not alone, that they are loved and that you won't let anything bad happen to them.

It is important to convey the message that it is all right to feel sad or frightened, to cry, to wonder, or to express feelings of anger or relief. Your acceptance of the child's feelings is a way of communicating your acceptance of her or him. Moreover, it lets your child know that such feelings are appropriate when someone important has been lost. In this way your child learns that grieving is normal.

Possibly, your child might experience your preoccupation with a baby who has died as a rejection of him or her, or as a message that he or she was lacking in some way: why else would you be so upset? Reassurance that the child is important, special, and loved often goes a long way toward alleviating these feelings. Similarly, the child may need reassurance that he or she has not lost his or her special place in the family. Verbal reassurance, physical closeness, and special time spent together are all ways of letting the child know that she or he is important to you.

Resist withdrawing into depression. Try not to leave your child's care to someone else or to minister to external needs while neglecting a more intimate relationship with him or her. Predictably, you are feeling exhausted, preoccupied, and depleted. You're not sure how much you have to give anyone. Nevertheless, make the effort to stay in close contact with your child during this stressful time. This will afford him maximum comfort and security and will also help keep you in communication. In addition, the comfort you derive both from seeing your child through this family crisis and from the closeness that you have created can be wonderfully healing for you as well.

FAMILY AND FRIENDS

You will find that in addition to coping with your own feelings and those of members of your immediate family, you will be affected by how other family members and friends respond to your loss. Not only will you be aware of their reactions to you, you will be mindful of your responses to them.

The loss of your baby probably has had an effect on the people around you. What your friends and family have in common is that they are likely to feel sad that your pregnancy ended as disastrously as it did. However, their personal reactions to your loss may vary tremendously, as does their capacity to communicate their feelings to you.

You may be especially grateful to some people for doing and saying all the "right" things and you may feel angry toward others for what they said or didn't say. Certain people "will never be forgotten" for their emotional support while others "will never be forgiven" for their lack of it.

Former patterns of communication with friends and family will probably continue during this time of crisis. If certain people have been supportive in the past, chances are you can depend on them now. Usually, there are a few people in your life whom you call first whenever something significant happens. They will probably be the first over to see you; caring for you as they do, they will want to be with you and share your grief. You will, no doubt, find that talking things over with people who care about you really helps.

REACTIONS TO YOUR LOSS

While generally the nature of your relationships will continue unchanged, you may be in for some surprises, both pleasant and unpleasant. Friends and family members may not be totally predictable in their reactions to your loss. Similarly, you may have some unexpected responses to others that may confuse you. Let us try to understand these unforeseen reactions and attempt to put them in perspective.

You may be pleasantly surprised to get a sympathetic call or note from a person you did not consider a close friend or relative — one whom you haven't spoken to in months, or even seen in years — who has heard about your loss through the grapevine. Such communication is welcome, since it is always nice to know there are people who understand. This contact may even eventually lead to a close friendship.

Many couples have found that after a pregnancy has been lost, friends, relatives, and acquaintances who have experienced similar losses are apt to share their own experiences with them. Often one learns of a friend's or relative's lost pregnancy only after having a loss yourself. Most people have found that being able to talk to other people who have also lost a pregnancy is a tremendous help to them. People who have themselves been through something similar will have a good understanding of what you are feeling. In addition, they will probably be able to give you invaluable advice and support. Beverly passed along this letter written by her mother-in-law, Isabel, after Beverly and her husband lost their second baby. Isabel had suffered both a stillbirth and an ectopic pregnancy before her son, Bob, was born. The couple found the letter a great source of comfort and encouragement. Isabel, more than anyone, knew the anguish they felt, and they turned to her constantly for support. As was typical of her, she was always consoling.

Dear Children,

Your phone call tonight informing me of the loss of your baby moved me so deeply that I must write. Beverly, dear, when you said, "It looks as if you won't be a grandmother," I'm so sorry. I must say that the thought hadn't occurred to me. All I could feel at the time was how desperately distressed you both must be.

Having lost two babies before you were born, Bob, I know the feeling of utter loss, the emptiness, the enormous disappointment you both must be experiencing now.

I mourn with you. My only words of comfort are that fortunately you are both young and well. Let us hope brighter times will come in the not too far future.

I love you both,
MOTHER

What may surprise and upset you will be the seeming insensitivity and lack of concern from people you thought cared about you. You may feel hurt and let down. You are probably confused by their inability to provide the support you need. You wonder, "Why doesn't she call me? Why do they pretend nothing has happened? Why do they tell me to just forget it and go on with my life?"

It is common to encounter relatives and friends who refuse to talk about the loss at all or who want to forget about the whole thing. Pregnancy loss is a time when people learn things about those close to them that may not be very pleasant to face — that some parents are self-centered, concerned with their own needs and unable to give to their grown children, for instance. With effort and attempts to communicate, some of these negative reactions might change. However, some attitudes may never change, and one must then accept this.

One woman told of her family's reaction at the time of her ectopic pregnancy: "They didn't know what to say, so they said nothing. Their silence was very painful to me and caused me ill feelings that will never heal. I wanted them to acknowledge our pain and they ignored it. They kept referring to it as my 'surgery' whenever they did bring it up. They just didn't know how to deal with it."

As we said earlier, individual reactions to your loss vary tremendously. Try to keep in mind that a person's reaction to you is based on his or her underlying personality and experiences. Also, that his reactions to you are a reflection of his own way of coping with things, as well as of his own life experiences. For example, one woman explains her sister-in-law's behavior the following way: "My sister-in-law was sympathetic and visited me when I was home, but the miscarriage occurred at an extremely stressful time for her — starting a new job — so she was preoccupied with that and had very little time for me."

Your loss may trigger feelings in friends and family members that cause them to be upset and confused. They may have a difficult time coping with their own painful feelings as well as with yours. In addition, they may be at a loss to know what to say to you. Rather than say the wrong thing, they may feel it best to say nothing at all. You may interpret their silence to mean they don't care when, in fact, they care so much they fear hurting you further.

On the other hand, you may find some people who don't understand what you are going through. If they have no interest in having children, they may not comprehend why you feel so badly. They have no sense of your yearning for a child, so they can't grasp your disappointment. Couples who have succeeded easily in having children and take pregnancy and birth for granted may not understand your frustration and pain, yet others with children may comprehend your grief completely. Although they had no problems, they fully appreciate the joys of parenthood. They are sensitive enough to feel hurt and disturbed that you have been denied what they find so fulfilling. They need only put themselves in your place and imagine the horror it would have been if they had lost their baby.

Another group of parents may react in a different way. They have children but are unhappy as parents. Some may be sorry they ever had children and feel that you are better off to have lost your baby. Their pregnancies might have been accidental, or regretted. These feelings are not easy to admit to oneself and even harder to confess to someone else, but they may be present in some of the people you know, and this may influence the way they deal with you.

Friends who are pregnant may worry that they, too, will lose their baby. Even a couple contemplating pregnancy may be fearful. When a friend or relative loses a baby, the saying "It can't happen to me" loses some of its credibility. Years after the birth of her son, one woman told her cousin: "Before you lost your baby, I never thought those things *really* happened. When I became pregnant, I worried constantly that my baby would die, as yours did. My fear was particularly strong in my eighth month, since your baby died then, so unexpectedly. I had a whole different way of thinking about my pregnancy because of what happened to you. I was terrified." A couple who is expecting a child may find it too anxiety-provoking to see you and may cope by avoiding you. This doesn't mean they are not sympathetic or don't care, but that they are scared it might happen to them and don't want to be reminded of the possibility.

Your pregnancy loss may evoke in others fear that might not be limited to issues regarding pregnancy. The death of your baby, although it was unborn, is a death nonetheless. Some people use denial and avoidance to cope with the issue of death. Hearing you discuss how badly you feel may be both painful and threatening for them. Your mourning may remind them that they and those around them are vulnerable to death at any time — they cannot control its inevitability. Rather than face these disconcerting feelings, they may stay away completely or avoid discussing your loss with you. It may be difficult for you to accept such avoidance behavior from family members and friends. There are times when our needs conflict with the needs of those we care about. Maybe there will be a change with time, and the relationship will survive, but it may not.

EXPECTANT GRANDPARENTS

Some reactions of family members may be based solely on the unique nature of family relationships. In many families, the parents of the couple who lost the baby were devastated by the news. It was painful to watch their children suffer and to know the tremendous impact of the loss on their lives. In addition, the loss of their grandchild-to-be was painful for them, because they, too, had been anticipating the new addition to the family. They, too, had fantasies and were terribly disappointed. To some, the child would have been their child as well — their second chance to be parents, particularly if they had no other grandchildren. In addition, the baby may have represented a new lease on life for them, or an exciting change, as they faced the onset of old age. Mothers often reexperience both their own pregnancies and their wish for a child when their daughters become pregnant. After the loss, they may feel personally deprived, aware of how the child would have touched their own life.

Because grandparents-to-be often experience a personal loss when their child's pregnancy fails, they may experience some of the same emotional reactions that their children are feeling — pain, sadness, emptiness, anger and disappointment. These feelings are intensified by the fact that their children are hurting. They mourn with their children and they mourn for themselves.

HELP OTHERS TO HELP YOU

Other people sometimes don't understand what they can do for you to help you feel better. Don't assume they understand the depths of your loss, particularly if they haven't been through the experience themselves.

It is best to assume that your friends and family may want to do the right thing but do not know what the right thing is. Not everyone instinctively knows what you want. The first thing to do is to figure out for yourself what you want from people, then tell them your wishes.

You may have friends or family members who are afraid to ask about your feelings. They may be trying to avoid opening a Pandora's box, while you would like nothing more than to pour your heart out. You may need to initiate the discussion. Give them a chance to be there for you. This is a time to strengthen bonds with friends and relatives.

If you are especially sensitive to the things people say to you, tell them if they are hurting your feelings. If hearing "It happened for the best" upsets you, let people know. They probably have put themselves in your place and are saying what they would like to hear. A simple explanation of how you are feeling should set things straight: "I understand you're trying to be helpful, but I can't accept the idea that it happened for the best at this time. It only makes me feel worse. I'm grieving for my lost baby."

There may be some practical things you would like your friends and family to do for you. It is likely they will be more than happy to help. Possibly you need help with shopping, cooking, or cleaning, or you may feel that you need to rest, or that you need time alone. If you have other children, you may need someone to help you with child care from time to time. Whenever possible tell people who wish to help you how they can be most helpful to you. They will feel better if they can do something for you, and chances are you will feel better, too.

IV

Planning for the Future ❧ ❧ ❧ ❧

Under the best of circumstances, it is extremely difficult to deal with the loss of a desired pregnancy. Hopes are shattered and faith in your own body may be badly damaged. In addition, you must face the frustration of not being able to control your destiny, whether on the level of being able to set a schedule for achieving certain life goals, or even for being able to have the things you want.

The loss of your pregnancy has probably caused a major disruption in your plans. From the moment you found out you were pregnant, all of your plans centered around the pregnancy and the expectation that you would have a baby.

You may have planned your career around the upcoming birth, stopped working or cut back in order to get ready for the baby. You may have made arrangements for a leave of absence from your job, or decided to stay at home indefinitely with your baby. If you have not been working, you may have modified your usual activities in anticipation of having a baby.

When you were pregnant, you may have bought or made maternity or baby clothes and picked out birth announcements. Friends and family may have worked away feverishly to have everything ready for your due date. You may have envisioned how "big" you would be by Thanksgiving, that you would feel the baby kick by your husband's birthday, and that you would be "waddling around" by the first of April.

Then, in one moment, all your dreams and plans were shattered. There was no baby, not this time.

You are faced with an awesome and overwhelming task. You must deal with your grief and at the same time reorient yourself to the reality of not being pregnant and not having the baby you yearn for.

It is not going to be easy to cope with the emptiness and pain; they will be with you for a long time. Try to accept that they cannot be erased.

How do you put together the pieces of your life when you are paralyzed with grief and unable to know what the future holds in store? There are no simple answers to this question. Each couple must travel the lonely road back from despair in their own time and in their own way. Each must confront many painful feelings, overcome them, and eventually lay them to rest. Then, and only then, will they be ready to go on with their lives.

The loss of your pregnancy has no doubt affected you emotionally, and perhaps physically as well. Because this has happened to you, decisions that you made in the past may no longer be desirable or feasible. Among the most important choices that will be facing you is whether you still want a child or whether you want to keep your family the size it already is. If you decide that you want a child, you must then ask yourself whether you wish to try to become pregnant again, if you wish to adopt, of if you would like to pursue both possibilities simultaneously. The decision that you reach should be based on many considerations, including what the chances are that you will be able to become pregnant, or that a new pregnancy will be successful. You must also assess whether you are feeling ready to cope with the stress of being pregnant again; what medical risks you may be facing; and what the risk is of producing a child with a serious genetic disorder. In addition, you need to think about how much you want to have a child; how long you are willing to wait to have a child; if adoption is a possible alternative for you; and how flexible you are about the type of child you would be willing to take.

After thinking about these issues, and discussing them between yourselves, with your physician, and, if indicated, with a geneticist or genetics counselor or a specialist in high-risk pregnancies, you must make a decision. You may decide to try again, even if the odds for success are not great, or the risk to you or your child is significant. Although there may be some possibility that you could have a successful pregnancy if you tried again, you may not be willing to take the emotional or physical risks involved. You may decide that you prefer to remain childless or to maintain your family at its present size, or you may elect to adopt. Possibly you do not feel ready to make any decision for a while. You may be feeling depleted and in need of time to recover before tackling something new, or you may be feeling too vulnerable to plunge into a pregnancy right now. The choice about how to proceed is a personal one.

10 ❧

Choosing to Try Again

Most of you will make the decision to try to become pregnant again. This is a successful coping mechanism because it has the potential to give you what you want most: a baby. Once you have made this decision you will need to think about how long you want to wait before trying to become pregnant. We suggest that you examine the following considerations.

MEDICAL CONSIDERATIONS

There is some controversy among physicians about what is the optimal time to wait before trying to conceive again. It is generally felt that the likelihood of miscarriage is diminished if conception is not attempted until the woman has had three normal menstrual periods. However, a minority of physicians feel that such a long time is not necessary, and that if the woman is anxious to become pregnant again, she may attempt conception after having one normal menstrual period. Since controversy exists about this matter, you will want to base your decision on your physician's recommendation, as well as on your own inclination.

Regardless of what time period is actually decided upon, you may be faced with the urge not to wait. A strong desire to become pregnant immediately may overshadow your rational decision. You may throw caution to the wind and attempt to become pregnant as soon as possible. Alternatively, you may choose to resist temptation because you want to do everything in your power to make your next pregnancy successful. Some couples choose to wait before trying again, because they believe that if they don't, and then lose their next pregnancy, they will blame themselves. This, too, should be taken into consideration in making your decision.

PSYCHOLOGICAL CONSIDERATIONS

There is some controversy about the length of time one should let pass before one is psychologically ready to try again. There are those who believe that a couple should wait six months to a year before conceiving or adopting. This recommendation is based on concern that unless they have sufficient time to mourn the child they lost, a second child may be regarded as a replacement. It is generally believed that in order for each child to be dealt with as a separate and unique individual, the parents' mourning process must be completed. Otherwise there is risk of contaminating the relationship with future children with unresolved feelings and fantasies about the child who was lost. It is also important for the couple to consider whether or not they feel ready to face trying again, and whether they feel ready to deal with the stress of another pregnancy.

We have found that the optimal time to wait before trying again is an individual matter and depends on one's own personality structure, past experiences, motivation to be a parent, and support network. It has been our experience that what is critical is that one has mourned one's loss, not how long a time period actually passes before a new pregnancy is attempted.

THE WAITING PERIOD

Most physicians recommend the use of a mechanical method of birth control (such as condoms, a diaphragm, or foam) during the waiting period. Like many couples, you may find it painful and ironic to have to use birth control at a time when you strongly desire to be pregnant. You may also find that mechanical methods of birth control are inconvenient and that they interrupt spontaneous lovemaking. Each time you make love you are faced with the decision of using or not using contraception. This conflict may trigger painful feelings all over again.

During the waiting period you will probably anticipate what it will be like when you begin trying to get pregnant. You may feel hopeful and optimistic, eagerly await each menstrual period, and count the days until you can try again. Or possibly you may feel anxious to try again, but extremely fearful that you will not be able to conceive. If you have a history of infertility, this fear may be intensified.

TRYING AGAIN

When the waiting is over and the time to try again finally arrives, you may find yourself in an emotional state you did not anticipate. You may have conflicting feelings: the fear of *not becoming* pregnant and the fear of *becoming* pregnant. In addition, the fears you had when you were waiting to try may be accentuated now that the possibility of pregnancy is closer at hand. You may be preoccupied with becoming pregnant to the exclusion of everything in your life. You may find yourself living by the menstrual cycle and you may find that your entire existence is focused on becoming pregnant. If you have had an infertility problem, you may discover that many of your feelings are familiar.

During the fertile time of the month you may find yourself obsessed with becoming pregnant. You may fantasize where the egg is each hour, not wanting to lose an opportunity to become pregnant. Now is the time to have intercourse whether or not you feel like it. You are motivated to have sex, not for pleasure but for procreation. This may lead to sexual difficulties such as refusal to "perform," performance anxiety, or decreased libido. As you approach the end of your cycle you may feel both anxious and hopeful that you won't have to go through another month of this. You may be preoccupied with searching for signs and symptoms of early pregnancy.

Marion was thirty-eight years old when she became pregnant for the first time. She had been trying for two years. She miscarried at nine weeks and decided to attempt another pregnancy four months later, partially because of her age. She told us that she was obsessed with becoming pregnant and that all else in her life had lost its meaning. She speaks of her behavior during this time: "Each month I spent one week constantly touching my breasts to see if they were sore like the first time I was pregnant and hoping they would hurt.

For several days before my period was due, I ran to the bathroom every hour, praying there would be no blood."

If your period arrives, you feel angry, frustrated, and in despair. The first day of your menstrual period is most likely to be the worst of the month. Another month has gone by without success, and you start to wonder if you'll ever get pregnant again.

The cycle repeats itself as you gear up for the next try. As ovulation approaches, you put aside your disappointment and get ready to try again.

BEING PREGNANT AGAIN

"Congratulations! You are pregnant." Those magic words! This is the moment you have been waiting for, and you feel ecstatic. After what have seemed to you like endless months of waiting, your prayers have been answered. You want to shout out your news; you feel like phoning up everyone you know to tell them. But you don't — something holds you back.

Better be cautious; better not tell anyone until you are sure, you tell yourself. Within minutes you discover that this pregnancy is simply not going to be like your first.

What makes this time different is that you have lost your innocence. This time you are aware of all the things that can go wrong. You know that if it happened once, it could happen again. Although you want to relax and enjoy being pregnant, anxiety keeps getting in your way. Sometimes the pregnancy feels like a nightmare, full of fear and remembrances of your previous pregnancy. Many women find that they are eternally vigilant — every twinge, pain, or cramp is noted, amplified, and feared.

We talked to Julie before the birth of her son. She was eight months pregnant. Even though her chances of carrying this baby to term were excellent, she was still suffering from the trauma of her first experience. She had lost her first baby a year earlier in her sixth month. No reason for the stillbirth was diagnosed. Julie described her constant state of fear: "The first six months of *this* pregnancy I was terrified. I kept dreaming of my labor and delivery, the doctor was saying, 'You're gonna lose it.' I dreaded going to the bathroom for fear there would be blood. I always felt reassured when my breasts were sore. I wanted this baby more than anything in the world, and because I wanted it so much, I felt sure that something would go wrong. At the beginning I spent endless hours imagining things that could go wrong — I would convince myself that I didn't have a chance. Every time I felt a twinge of pain I would feel hysterical inside. I lost my ability to tell which pains were normal and which weren't — everything felt the same to me — anything could mean the end of all of my hopes.

"I must have called my doctor a dozen times to tell him about one concern or another. Usually he would tell me not to worry. However, if I was really frantic he would always see me. Luckily, he never found anything to worry about, and I was always able to leave his office somewhat reassured. Unfortunately, my feelings of well-being never lasted very long. Within a few days, I would find something else to worry about.

"I think I almost drove my husband crazy. Sometimes it got so bad that I would convince him that there really was something wrong with the baby. Those times were the worst. Even though I am in my eighth month, I'm still terrified. I can't forget what I went through and I live in constant fear of it happening again this time. I probably won't rest until the baby is in my arms."

Even when things do go well, it may be hard to enjoy being pregnant. This can be a frustrating experience. You wish you could be as blissfully oblivious as other pregnant women. You yearn to be able to enjoy being pregnant, the way other women do — it doesn't seem fair to have this spoiled also. Unfortunately, if you have ever had the experience of losing a pregnancy, pregnancy probably will never again be a state of bliss for you. With luck, there will be many happy moments. It is likely that there will also be some tense or anxious ones, not because anything will necessarily go wrong, but because sometimes it is hard not to imagine the worst. Some women have likened the experience of losing a pregnancy to the way they felt the first time someone they knew died. Before someone you actually know dies, you know about death, but it doesn't really have an impact on you. Death is something that happens to people out there, not to anyone in your world. Beforehand, death is an abstract concept, without any real meaning. Afterward, life feels incredibly fragile, and you realize how very vulnerable you are. The same seems to hold true for pregnancy.

Before you actually lost a pregnancy, you probably knew that some pregnancies were unsuccessful. However, if you were like most women, you probably didn't give this much thought. Since it happened to you, your fear of losing a pregnancy is probably much greater. Rationally you know that most pregnancies are successful; still, it is difficult not to feel anxious. Once you lose your innocence, there is no way of getting it back. You have been changed by your experience, and will never be the same again.

A Precious Pregnancy

If you have lost a pregnancy, it is doubtful that you will ever take being pregnant for granted. This has both its good side and its more problematic side. On the positive side, it is likely that you will truly value being pregnant and will have an appreciation of the miracle that is unfolding inside you. This would not have been as possible had you not experienced the pain you have been through. For you, pregnancy will never be just something that is going on in your body while the rest of you is occupied with more important things. Similarly, there is little danger that you will miss one precious moment, that even the smallest new development will pass unnoticed, or that you will fail to set aside time to appreciate the experience fully.

On the problematic side is the anxiety that almost always accompanies a particularly "precious" pregnancy. This is no ordinary pregnancy for you. This is the pregnancy that you have been hoping for and dreaming of. If you are like most women who have once lost a pregnancy, you are not about to do the slightest thing to endanger it. Not for you the advice that "pregnancy is a natural state; you need not curtail your usual activities, unless they are particularly strenuous or dangerous." The moment you find out that you are pregnant, you feel like a fragile vessel carrying an even more fragile cargo. Rationally you know that a normal pregnancy is quite impervious to bumps, jumps, and even falls. However, you may decide that although this might be true for other women, you prefer to play it safe. If you have questions about what activities are permissible, ask your physician for his opinion. If he does not feel that you need to restrict your activities, your personal preference can be your guide. You should do only what you feel psychologically and physically comfortable doing. Some women find that their anxiety pervades every aspect of their lives. One otherwise undaunted woman felt that danger was everywhere and became phobic during the pregnancy that followed a stillbirth. More common is the experience of being anxious and hypervigilant about the pregnancy. If one's anxiety feels overwhelming, it is a good idea to speak to one's physician about it. He or she may be able to offer reassurance, more frequent visits, or more extensive monitoring than usual. Referral to a counselor may also be helpful.

Expecting Too Much

"This is the pregnancy you have been looking forward to, and now that it is a reality, you'd better enjoy every moment of it." "This is a precious moment in your life, and you'd better cherish it." Thoughts like these are commonly experienced by pregnant women who have lived through infertility, losing a pregnancy, or both. Noble sentiments; however, not totally realistic. Pregnancy, under the best of circumstances, can have its less appealing side. Fatigue, nausea, and vomiting are common in the first trimester, while a variety of aches and pains, exhaustion, urinary frequency, and trouble getting around often bother even the heartiest of souls during the third trimester. Not you, however; you are supposed to be grateful that you are pregnant, and you don't have the right to complain about any part of it. If a complaint manages to sneak out, you feel guilty — after all this was what you wanted, wasn't it? After wanting to be pregnant so badly, you probably feel that it is unreasonable of you to have negative feelings about any part of it.

Often when we very much want something that is not immediately available to us, we create fantasies of what it would be like to have our wish come true. These fantasies are usually a highly idealized, and therefore unrealistic, version of the real thing. The problem is that often the real thing is not quite as good as the fantasy: that is, it is not as good as you imagined it would be. When we imagine what being pregnant will be like, we think of a rounded belly, full breasts, ourselves proudly wearing maternity clothes, and a beaming husband. Endless mornings of nausea, sleepiness, and anxiety just aren't what dreams are made of, yet for many women, this is what pregnancy is apt to be like.

A word of caution: in the same way that your fantasies of what pregnancy would be like may have led you to have unrealistic expectations about the experience, and of yourself as a pregnant woman, your fantasies about what it will be like to have a baby and to be a mother may leave you ill prepared for dealing with the less glorious aspects of that experience. Both pregnancy and motherhood can be pleasurable and fulfilling; they can also be difficult and frustrating, especially when you feel that there is something wrong with you for feeling that you should not have any negative feelings.

Holding Back

Fear of losing another baby inhibits many couples from emotionally investing in the next pregnancy. They know that loss can happen again, and so try to protect themselves in case it does. Often, they allow themselves little, if any, bonding with the baby during pregnancy. Some say that "holding back" was their way of protecting themselves from feeling completely devastated should this pregnancy also fail.

Even when things go well, and the pregnancy progresses normally, it may be difficult to invest your love and hope. Julie, whom we spoke about a while earlier, found it difficult to allow herself to feel attached to her unborn child, not because she didn't love it, but because she wanted it so badly. "I never really let myself enjoy being pregnant. I held my feelings back the entire time. I tried not to let myself think about a baby — in fact, I almost managed to disconnect being pregnant from having a baby. It was almost as if, if I relaxed and allowed myself to believe that I really was going to have a child, something would come along and take it all away. I know that I was protecting myself from feeling too disappointed had anything gone wrong. Last time I was so devastated that, no matter what, I didn't want to ever feel that way again. I guess that my husband felt the same way, because we seemed to have an unspoken agreement that this time we would not let our hopes grow. I think that in some ways we both were emotionally frozen throughout the pregnancy."

Julie and her husband decided not to let their friends and family know about the pregnancy until her sixth month was completed. They felt that they would be tempting fate to announce it before then. They also felt that they would be less disappointed if the pregnancy was lost before everyone knew about it. Julie's reluctance to let people know is not unusual; many couples who have lost pregnancies choose to do the same. Some say that they felt too vulnerable to let other people know, others felt that by not telling they could protect families and friends from feeling disappointed. Even couples who do not hold off telling others as long as Julie did, often wait until the end of the third month to let people know, since the major danger of losing the pregnancy is over by then.

Although there is usually no rational cause for concern, many women find that they are unable to enjoy their pregnancies until they have passed the month when their first babies died. Often after this point their anxiety subsides. Many hold off telling people that they are pregnant and wearing maternity clothes until the "magic" month has passed. Charlotte, the relieved mother of a beautiful three-month-old girl, reflected back on her most recent pregnancy. Her first baby died at the seventh month for unknown reasons.

"I was very scared during my first seven months that I would lose my baby again. I took extra good care of myself: resting, eating well. After I passed my seventh month I decided to be happy and enjoy being pregnant. I had gotten robbed the first time and was determined to make it up. I made my mind up that I would deal with the loss if and when it happened.

"Early on, my husband and doctor were the only people who knew I was pregnant again. I did not tell anyone until I was obviously showing or they asked outright. I was too afraid this one would die too and I'd have to explain it all over again. I held off buying maternity clothes as long as I could, then I bought them piece by piece. I didn't want to buy a lot of things and then have no reason to wear them. I had thrown away all my old maternity clothes after I lost my last baby because I couldn't bear to look at them. I felt it would be bad luck to wear them this time.

"Only after my seventh month passed did I feel safe enough to buy any baby clothes or start furnishing the nursery. I even started to believe that I was really going to have a baby."

Waiting for the Results of Amniocentesis

Couples who anticipate having to have an amniocentesis often find themselves unable to feel a sense of relief until they have obtained the test results and learned that all is well. Amniocentesis is a procedure that has been available in recent years for determining whether the fetus has any one of a number of genetic or metabolic conditions. It is usually recommended for all women who are thirty-five or older. This is because women over the age of thirty-five have a significantly increased risk of producing a child with Down syndrome (also known as mongolism or trisomy 21). Women under thirty have approximately one chance in 1,500 of having a child with Down syndrome. The incidence of this disease increases markedly with the mother's age, so that the chance that a woman between the ages of thirty and thirty-four will have an afflicted child is 1 in 750. Between thirty-five and thirty-nine the incidence is about 1 in 300, and between forty and forty-four it is approximately 1 in 80.

Amniocentesis is also recommended to parents of any age if they have produced a child with a genetic defect, if they have produced a child who has an inherited metabolic disorder, such as Tay-Sachs disease or Gaucher's disease, or if they themselves are either carriers of these conditions, have a family history of inherited disease, or are themselves affected. For example, a couple whose family is known to carry a sex-linked chromosomal disorder such as hemophilia or Duchenne muscular dystrophy may wish to have an amniocentesis performed.

The actual procedure in an amniocentesis is very simple. Sometime between the fifteenth and seventeenth week of gestation, a procedure known as ultrasound scanning, which uses high-frequency sound waves to visualize the fetus, the placenta, and the amniotic cavity, is used to pinpoint these structures. Using local anesthesia, a needle is inserted through the pregnant woman's abdomen into the amniotic sac, and a small amount of yellowish amniotic fluid is drawn off. This fluid contains some fetal cells. Samples of the amniotic fluid are then sent to the laboratory for study. The fetal cells are incubated, and when they have reproduced sufficiently, they are subjected to a number of tests. It takes from one to three weeks until there are a sufficient number of cells so that tests can be done. The amniotic fluid itself is analyzed for the presence of a specific protein, alpha-fetoprotein, unusually high concentrations of which can indicate that the fetus has an open neural tube defect.

In indicated, other specific tests can be done to determine whether the fetus has any one of several biochemical abnormalities, which could cause a metabolic disease (for instance, lack of the enzyme hexosaminidase A indicates presence of Tay-Sachs disease), or whether an inherited sex-linked disease such as hemophilia can be diagnosed.

Lastly, cells are isolated from the tissue culture, specially stained, and then viewed under electron microscope, to determine whether the fetus has any chromosomal abnormalities, such as Down syndrome.

The weeks between the time when the amniocentesis is done and the final tests are completed are difficult ones for most couples. The test results will indicate if, as far as could be ascertained, the fetus is normal or whether a defective fetus has been discovered. In the latter situation, which occurs in a minority of cases, it is still early enough in the pregnancy for a safe therapeutic abortion to be performed.

Because the continuation of the pregnancy is contingent on the outcome of the amniocentesis, many couples find it difficult to invest themselves in the pregnancy until they are certain that it will not have to be interrupted. One veteran of two amniocenteses described feeling as if her emotions were suspended until she learned that each fetus was normal. Only after obtaining the report indicating that all was well was she able to let herself form an attachment to her future child. This woman's experience is fairly typical. No matter how optimistic one is, it is the rare couple that does not breathe a sigh of relief when the test results come back indicating that no abnormalities were found. For more information about prenatal diagnosis see chapter 5.

WHEN YOUR BABY ARRIVES

Parents who have lost a pregnancy often find that although the birth of a child eases their pain greatly, it does not erase it entirely.

They discover that there is no starting afresh, that the memory of what they have been through stays with them and affects them in many ways.

Commonly, couples who have experienced the loss of a pregnancy protect themselves from becoming too attached to subsequent pregnancies. One effect of this may be that for them the bonding process to their child begins at birth, rather than beforehand. Also, since they may not have allowed themselves to think very much about what it would be like to be a parent or to take care of a child, they may find themselves less psychologically prepared for their new role than are couples who have spent the pregnancy anticipating what would be expected of them. As a consequence, they may find that for a brief time after their baby's birth they can't quite believe that they actually have a child and that they are its parents. These feelings are experienced by many new parents and are nothing to be concerned about. Fortunately love develops quickly, as do caretaking skills, and within a few days or weeks it feels as if the baby has always been theirs.

It is also likely that the baby born of a "precious pregnancy" will be a very precious baby. It is to be hoped that this will only heighten your delight in your new child: this is your "miracle" child, the child you feared might never happen, and everything about him or her will probably feel quite special. It is also possible that the "specialness" of this child for you may make you feel overly concerned about his or her wellbeing or about your parenting ability.

People who have always had a predisposition to worry tend to be particularly vulnerable to this type of anxiety. A recent encounter with the cruelty of fate seems to reinforce their feelings of vulnerability: they fear that if something bad has happened to them once, it could happen again. While this fear is understandable, it is important to remember that just because you feel particularly vulnerable doesn't mean that you actually are. Most couples find that as time passes their anxiety gradually lessens. If you find that this is not so for you, counseling may be useful in helping you put the past in perspective, so that you can more fully enjoy being a parent.

It is also important to keep in mind that even the most special and long-awaited baby may at times be less than a total delight. There is a tendency among parents who have lost a pregnancy to feel that they are being ungrateful if they are ever tired, overworked, or short-tempered. After all, this is the baby they have been looking forward to for so long — what's wrong with them, they ask themselves, for sometimes feeling exhausted or upset? While it is normal to feel that not all aspects of being a parent are pleasurable, parents who have experienced pregnancy loss tend not to give themselves permission to have anything other than positive feelings. As a result, they often feel guilty and inadequate, although there is no real reason for feeling that way. This attitude may be compounded when friends and family members are insensitive to what the new parents are experiencing, and when they add their overblown expectations to the couple's own.

There is a tendency in our society to believe that a lost pregnancy can be replaced by a new one and that the scars that one develops when one loses a pregnancy are eradicated by the birth of a new baby. Most couples find that their experience is not quite so simple. Some couples may find that the birth of a child reopens old wounds, because it so vividly reminds them of what they had lost. While the birth of a child goes a long way toward alleviating the pain they feel, it does not do away with it entirely. There will always be feelings of regret at what could have been, as well as painful memories of what they had been through.

11 🎋

Choosing Childlessness

Once upon a time you made the decision to have children. When you made this decision, chances are that you assumed that if you wanted to have children you would be able to without difficulty. When things did not work out as you planned, you were forced to reconsider the options available to you.

The decision to remain childless comes about in different ways for different couples. Some couples discover that while they were willing to go ahead with having a child if it could be done easily, they were not willing to make the effort to have one if it meant enduring an infertility evaluation and medical treatment; the physical, emotional, and financial costs of continuing to try; the frustration and pain of enduring multiple losses; the risk of producing a child with a serious genetic disorder; or the effort to pursue adoption.

Some couples have found that the experience of being pregnant and losing a pregnancy has helped them recognize that childbearing was not for them. One or both partners may have found that they experienced doubts or negative feelings during the pregnancy. We picture pregnancy as a time of excitement and happiness, but it can also be a time of stress and uncertainty if one partner or both have doubts about whether they want to have children. The woman may find that being pregnant brings into focus many apprehensions. She may fear that if she has a child she will lose her freedom, or she may feel that having a child will bring about a drastic change in her responsibilities, whether she becomes a homemaker or continues working. She may feel she has to give up quite a lot in order to rear a child and may be unsure if she wants to make that commitment. The man may also be sensitive to the responsibility a child will bring, as well as to the change in lifestyle that having a child will bring about. He may be concerned that he will come second to a child in his wife's affections, or he may worry about the financial obligations involved in raising a child.

Sometimes couples choose to remain childless because they are unable to produce their own biological child, although they would have liked to; and one or both partners do not wish to adopt. When partners are in agreement about what they want, things usually work out well. More problematic are situations where one spouse wishes to adopt and the other does not wish to. This latter situation may leave one or both partners feeling angry, frustrated, or depressed, and when unresolved may cause major marital problems or even the breakup of the marriage.

Other couples remain childless, although they would like to have a child and would happily adopt one, either because they were not accepted by an agency, because they were not eligible to adopt the kind of child they were hoping for, because they were unable to find a child that they could adopt privately, or because private adoption is illegal in their state.

Childfree living can be a positive choice; as such it can be both satisfying and rewarding. Increasing numbers of couples are choosing not to have children. Couples who have made this choice feel that it affords them many advantages.

The couple who does not have children can choose to live life free of many of the constraints that influence couples with children. They can live and work in ways that suit themselves, but that might not be compatible with the needs of a child. Choices vary from options such as working long hours, pursuing a demanding career, or returning to school to earn a degree, all of which can be done with less trouble without a child than with one, to such unconventional options as pursuing work that one loves but that does not pay well, or traveling to remote areas of the globe for long or short periods of time. In almost every realm of their lives the couple without children has more freedom than do couples with children. For the most part they need pay attention to their own needs alone. This can mean going out to a movie or away for the weekend without making complicated arrangements, sleeping late without interruption, or having free time available for sports, visiting with friends, being together, or just doing nothing.

In addition, the couple who does not have children need provide financially only for themselves, and so may enjoy a larger share of whatever economic resources are available to them than would be the case if they had a child to feed, clothe, and shelter, not to mention to send to college. Inflation has made it difficult for the average family to get by with one salary; as a consequence many couples are choosing to have both partners work outside the home. In many areas child-care services do not meet the need for them, and when available are often quite costly. Without this support a couple's ability to both work and raise children may be severely compromised, perhaps making it necessary to choose between the two. When one adds up the cost of raising a child to the age of eighteen in the United States, estimated as costing over $100,000 in 1991, not counting the cost of college, it is not difficult to see why, for many couples, having children is a major economic burden.

In recent years, as women have entered the labor force in increasing numbers, many have found that their primary satisfaction could be derived from work, and that they neither needed nor wanted the added responsibility of having a child. Similarly, as women have been accepted into professional schools and career training programs in ever-increasing numbers and the possibilities for having a successful career have expanded, more women are electing to pursue career choices that either preclude entirely or make very difficult having a child.

Choosing not to have children of one's own need not mean that one must live a life without children. There are many ways for those who desire contact with children to bring this about. Teaching has long been a way for people who enjoy being with children to play a meaningful part in their lives. Working in a school as a nurse, maintenance person, dietitian, or secretary can yield similar benefits. So too can volunteer work with hospitalized, institutionalized, bedridden, or handicapped children, whose lives could be greatly improved by a relationship with a caring adult. Leading a Girl Scout or Boy Scout troop, being a Big Brother or Big Sister to a child, befriending neighborhood children, volunteering at a day-care center or becoming a special aunt or uncle to a niece or nephew are other possible ways to enrich your own life, as well as the lives of those who are lucky enough to have you for a friend.

One can choose to have as much or as little contact with children as one desires. Being foster parents to several children can totally fill your life; working for a cause that will ultimately benefit children can be far less time-consuming, but enormously gratifying, nonetheless. In short, the possibilities for having children in your life are many. The world is full of children to share and to love even if you don't bear or adopt your own.

As social pressure to conform to one acceptable lifestyle decreases, more and more people are exploring new alternatives. Child-free marriage is slowly and steadily gaining public acceptance as traditional ideas about what constitutes a family are expanded. The couple who chooses not to have children need no longer hide in the closet. Increasingly, groups such as ZPG (Zero Population Growth) and National Alliance for Optional Parenthood are serving as both a support group and as an advocate for couples who choose to remain childless.

The following is a description of one couple's route to choosing childlessness.

"After four years of trying to conceive and then two miscarriages, my husband and I decided to quit trying, but we hadn't given up on the idea of raising children. We had been through infertility testing and had conceived both times through artificial insemination (with my husband Steve's sperm). The problem was that my cervical mucus was hostile to Steve's sperm. We were very excited with the first pregnancy and crushed when it ended at about three months. We became less excited over the second pregnancy — I miscarried a week after the pregnancy test, at two and a half months.

"After the second loss, I kept telling myself we could try again, that there was hope, but I was also afraid of more disappointment. My age, thirty-eight, was uppermost in my mind — we couldn't keep trying for years on end. And the years of ups and downs of trying and hoping were taking a toll. I was edgy, easily depressed, and Steve, who had always been very patient and calm, was irritable. About a month after the second miscarriage, we had a long talk about our feelings and coping or lack of coping with our situation. "Do we really want to stay on this roller coaster?" Steve asked. I started to cry at the thought of giving up, but I had to admit that I longed to return to our normal life. My life had become centered on getting pregnant. I worked as a legal secretary, but felt I was only marking time until I could become a full-time mother. It was hard to face the fact that we might not have a child, as we had dreamed for so long. Steve and I agreed that night that we would think about other possibilities — adoption and childlessness. We had both been married previously and neither Steve nor I had children from those marriages. We realized we were getting old to have children and after seven years of marriage, a baby would be a big adjustment.

"I wasn't ready to give up entirely, though, and started looking into adoption. We went to an information meeting on adoption held by our county's social service department and found that only older children, not infants, were available. We felt inadequate to cope with a six-year-old who had lived in various foster homes. We felt discouraged. Then I contacted adoption agencies and heard there was a three- to five-year wait. Adoption didn't seem a good alternative for us — at our age we felt we couldn't wait and we doubted whether agencies would even accept our application. Wouldn't they be more likely to place babies with thirty-year-olds?

"We pondered adoption for a number of weeks and gradually decided against pursuing it. Then we just drifted for a while, several months at least, only occasionally discussing our quandary. I still wanted to be around kids, and a few months later an opportunity arose. Our church needed an elementary Sunday School teacher, so I volunteered. That was over a year ago. Steve helps with the class of about twenty youngsters, and we enjoy it very much.

"Over the last year since we decided to think about other possibilities than having our own children, we have become more relaxed. Our acceptance of our loss of our dream to have children was gradual. The reality of the situation slowly seeped in.

"My work means much more to me now and I'm taking classes to become a paralegal assistant. I'm developing a positive attitude about not having children, though there still is a pang at times.

"We have a good life together and are happier now that the stress of trying to conceive is gone. Nearly every Saturday or Sunday we go hiking, sometimes alone and sometimes with a club we belong to. We've found that our life is full."

12 ❧

Deciding to Adopt

If you are not able to conceive, if you are unable to carry a pregnancy successfully to term, or if you are unwilling to attempt another pregnancy because of genetic difficulties or because of either the physical or the emotional risk involved, and if you strongly desire to have a child and to experience parenthood, adoption is worth considering.

Perhaps the most significant aspect of the decision to adopt is that it is a "decision." Adoption is not the automatic, obvious way for most couples to fill the empty cradle in the nursery. Couples do not adopt by merely leading their normal lives and leaving things up to nature. In order for an adoption to happen, one must make a concerted effort to bring it about.

The process by which one decides whether or not to pursue adoption and the factors influencing the timing of this process are different for each couple. In part, how one proceeds is determined by where one begins. The couple who is certain that they will never be able to bear their own child may see adoption as offering them their only chance for having a child in their lives, whereas the couple who still has the potential ability to produce their own biological child, despite several unsuccessful pregnancies, may see adoption as an option for the future, rather than something they wish to consider for the present. The couple who has always considered adopting a child will find the idea less foreign than will the couple who has never considered the possibility. Most couples consider adopting a child when their own attempts at having a child have been unsuccessful. However, not everyone draws the line in the same place. Some couples are able to keep trying and to feel optimistic about their chances of success, despite many losses, while others decide to give up trying to have their own child after one or two unsuccessful pregnancies.

Each couple has to figure out when to begin the adoption process. This decision is easier for those who know that they are unable to have children. They are more likely to begin immediately after deciding that they wish to adopt.

On the other hand, couples who have experienced one or more unsuccessful pregnancies may still have the ability, albeit theoretical, to produce a child themselves. This group faces the most complex decision, since, as is so often true in life, they must base their deliberations on supposition rather than on fact. If four pregnancies have been unsuccessful, who is to say that the same will or will not hold true for the fifth pregnancy? When does it make sense to stop trying? Would one more try result in the birth of a much-desired child? If you have had one ectopic pregnancy, will the second pregnancy be different? Unfortunately, there is no way of predicting what the answers to these questions will be.

Since it is not possible to read the future, whatever decision is made must be based on either intuition, an overriding preference, or on a careful assessment of one's situation. If you have an intuitive sense of how to proceed, or if you *know* how you want to go about becoming parents, your path is before you. If, however, you are uncertain about whether or not you are ready to adopt, it may be helpful to weigh the following factors. First, with the help of your physician you should try to assess the likelihood that you will be able to carry a pregnancy successfully to term, and produce a healthy child. As one would guess, the prognosis for a successful pregnancy is different for the couple who has had a long history of fetal deaths and for the couple who has produced two children before having a single miscarriage. Your prognosis is dependent not only on your reproductive history; whether or not the cause of pregnancy loss has been determined may be of importance. If a treatable cause has been found, the odds of success may be different than if no cause has been found. Similarly, your current state of health needs to be taken into account in determining the prognosis for future pregnancies. Since some chronic diseases predispose to fetal loss, the woman who has such a condition needs to know if her current condition will negatively influence the outcome of a pregnancy.

Your age and that of your spouse are another factor that needs to enter into your decision-making process. If you are young, you have many years before you in which to keep trying before your biological time clock runs out. On the other hand, if you are in your late thirties or your forties and have been trying for years to have a child without success, it is doubtful, though not impossible, that several more years of trying will bring success.

In addition, if you would like to be able to apply to an adoption agency, your age at the time you apply may determine both whether or not the agency considers you eligible and what type of placement they would consider you eligible for. Since the upper age limit that most agencies consider suitable for an infant placement is somewhere around forty years, you increase your chance of being successful if you apply before you reach this age.

Other factors to weigh in deciding whether or not to adopt or to attempt another pregnancy are whether a pregnancy would subject you to significant physical risk and/or whether a pregnancy is likely to result in the birth of a congenitally defective child. A woman who has narrowly escaped death when her tube burst may not be anxious to tempt fate. Similarly, women with medical conditions that increase in severity during pregnancy may well be inclined to avoid further problems. So, too, the couple who has given birth to a child with a congenital defect, especially if the presence of the defect cannot be determined prenatally.

Some couples give up on trying to have a biological child and decide to adopt for other reasons. The wear and tear of years of trying may be significant, as may the feelings of disappointment and discouragement that result from it. It is not uncommon to feel that you just couldn't stand losing another pregnancy — that one more loss would do you in. Related to this is the desire for certainty that most couples have. Living with uncertainty can take its toll. In addition, coping with an uncertain future, especially when your desire for a child is strong, can be extremely stressful. Deciding to adopt is one way of eliminating the uncertainty that results from depending on one's own erratic biology.

The most important factor that leads many to adopt is the urgent desire to have a child. As one couple expressed this motivation: "We have lost valuable years, years when we would have liked to have had a child in our lives. I guess we could keep on trying to have our own, but who knows if we ever will, and even if we did eventually, who is to predict how many years from now that will be. I guess neither of us are willing to take the chance that someday we might be successful."

One of the first things that most couples who have considered adoption realize is that adopting a child is not the same as producing one's own biological child. In order to determine whether adoption is right for you, you should ask yourself how you feel about some of the differences. Among the gratifications an adopted child cannot offer are the experience and satisfaction of biologically creating a human being, the ability to enhance your marriage by producing a child with your spouse, the fulfillment of experiencing pregnancy and childbirth, and the security of being equal to and like your friends and relatives who have had their own biological children.

You must be able to come to terms with the loss of these "biological benefits" before you can completely accept adoption as an alternative. It is not easy for those of us who have spent our entire lives expecting that someday we would produce a child of our own to give up that goal.

Nevertheless, couples who recognize that their goal is to have a child in their lives, and who feel that this desire overshadows their need for a biological connection, are able to find fulfillment by adopting a child.

The realization that parenthood is one's primary goal does not, however, end the decision-making process. Other valid and important questions must be answered before an intelligent choice can be made. For example, the question "Can I love an adopted child?" must be confronted. One must examine one's need to love another, and understand it thoroughly, before one can comfortably and unambivalently say "Yes." It is also necessary to ask yourself what type of child you prefer, and how flexible you are able to be about what you could accept. Could you love an older child, a handicapped child, or a child of a different race, or is the only type of child you would consider adopting one that is similar to what you would have produced?

Another area that is worth some thought is how you feel about the "adoptive relationship." Are you worried that your child will not love you, because you did not give birth to him or her? Are you concerned about how to tell your child about his or her origins? Are you fearful that the child's biological parents will show up on your doorstep one day, or that your child will seek them out? Do you feel that your child's biological parents, whether personally known or anonymous, will feel like potential rivals to you?

If you find these issues disturbing, you may find that it is helpful to put your fears in context. The concerns that you as a potential adoptive parent are experiencing all have their counterpart in the kinds of concerns that biological parents deal with. Thus, your concern that your child's love will be taken away by his biological parents really raises a question all parents must face . . . namely, will my child continue to love me when he's older, or will he reject me? Biology does not create love. Similarly, your worry about what to tell your adoptive child about his origins has its analogue in an issue which all humans must deal with. When one sets out to produce a baby one is dealing with a genetic process that is quite random. There is no way of determining which egg will unite with which sperm, to form a particular embryo, and eventually a particular child. One's genetic history is largely accidental. There is no guarantee that one's child will get your "good" qualities. It might just as easily inherit your less desirable traits or, worse, those of your least favorite relative! If this rationale fails to convince you that your adoptive child is no worse biologically for not coming from you, it should at least dispel another preadoptive parental concern: that an adopted child will not be as "good" as what you could have produced.

Lastly, in assessing whether or not adoption is for you, you must also determine whether you are willing to expend the time, energy, and financial resources it often takes. It is widely acknowledged that obtaining a child for adoption and legalizing an adoption require herculean efforts. This is when your motivation and emotional acceptance of adoption are tested, for it is rare than an adoptable child falls out of the sky and into one's home. Couples must look at alternatives — childlessness, no more children, or a total reliance upon their own reproductive organs. At some point, those who choose adoption simply refuse to be denied or scared off and determine that they will do whatever it takes.

Sometimes the effort required is considerable. As the various means of adopting are explored, decisions must again be made and new fears overcome. Unfortunately, no matter how motivated a couple may be, many are sidetracked for years by a lack of correct information. Because laws, agency rules, and sources of babies vary and are all subject to change, the most successful couples leave no stone unturned, scrutinize all sources of information and refuse to accept "no" for an answer.

Part of the decision to adopt a child is the acceptance of the fact that, like producing a child biologically, it is not necessarily going to be easy. It may cost time, energy, and money. It may cause frustration, embarrassment, and sadness. It is good practice for the tough side of parenthood.

Practical questions influence whether and by what means a couple pursues adoption. Some couples are immediately attracted to children who are handicapped, older, part of a group of siblings, and/or not of their race. Other couples want only what they had hoped to produce themselves: a healthy infant of their own general appearance. Some couples prefer an agency-arranged placement because it provides the most legal safeguards from a change of heart by the biological parents during the pendency of the adoption. Other couples may choose private adoption, either because they are unwilling to wait the years it takes for an agency placement, because they prefer to have as much information about or to know the birth parents as well as possible, or because they were judged ineligible for consideration by the agencies to which they applied. State laws that either allow or forbid private adoption also dictate the course of action a couple can take. The decision to adopt is, then, really a two-step process: first, the decision that adoption is desired must be reached; second, after an investigation of available resources, the method of making it happen has to be determined.

AGENCY ADOPTION

The most common and accepted way in which prospective adoptive parents seek to find a child is through a licensed domestic adoption agency, which acts as a socially approved intermediary whose task it is to distribute a limited supply of children to those who seem to it most suitable.

The average wait for a healthy newborn in the United States is currently somewhere between five and seven years. The situation for hard-to-place children — those older than eight years, minority children, children who are part of a sibling group, and children with physical, intellectual, or emotional handicaps — is generally less discouraging. This is because there are more children in these categories available for placement, as well as fewer prospective parents whose first choice is a hard-to-place child. Both the selection criteria that agencies use and the length of time you should expect to wait before being given a child reflect these realities.

In order for you to make your decision about whether or not you wish to pursue adoption through an agency, it is important that you know both some of the advantages and some of the disadvantages of selecting this route.

The primary reason that leads couples to adopt through an agency is that agencies are still a good source of children. Equally important to many is the fact that agency adoption affords them the best legal safeguards. Before an agency will place a child in your home, the mother and the father, if known, are required to sign papers relinquishing the child. This relinquishment is final unless obtained under false pretenses or under duress. Once the child is placed in your home by an agency, you can relax in the knowledge that the parents have forfeited their rights and cannot at any time change their minds about this and successfully seek to reclaim their child. An additional plus is that the agency acts as go-between in the transaction between biological and adoptive parents, thereby assuring anonymity for both. The agency also attempts to investigate both the health and backgrounds of the biological parents and the health of the child it places with you, so that you can be as informed as possible about what difficulties you might encounter. Lastly, agencies locate the babies they place, thereby requiring of the prospective adoptive parents far less initiative than if they were to search for a child on their own.

There are several reasons why agency adoption is not the route taken by all those who seek to adopt. Foremost, agency adoption, particularly of healthy newborns, is highly competitive. The selection criteria that agencies use are designed to select those individuals who they believe will best be able to meet the needs of the child waiting to be adopted. These criteria are set and administered by each individual agency. This means that if they do not see you as meeting their criteria for successful adoptive parents, you will either be discouraged from applying at all, or in less clearcut situations you may be rejected once your application is reviewed. Some of the criteria that agencies use in making their selection will be detailed later.

Some individuals or couples who might be found to be suitable candidates by an agency also choose to look elsewhere for a child. Some feel that the entire application process and home study is an invasion of privacy. Others feel resentful that because they are infertile they have to prove that they would be suitable parents. The long waiting period for a child is still another deterrent. Those who prefer to search for a child themselves, and those who feel that they want to get to know the biological mother or parents directly may also find that an agency adoption does not meet their needs.

Finding an Agency

Let us suppose that after weighing the pros and cons you have decided that you would like to adopt through an agency. The first thing that you have to do after making this decision is to find an agency. If you live near a large city there are probably a number of agencies from which to choose. There are two types of agencies: public and private. Public agencies are supported by taxes and run by the city or county department of welfare or social services. Generally, the fees you would be expected to pay are lowest in a public agency. Private agencies can be either nonsectarian or affiliated with and financed by a specific religious group. The latter specializes in adoptions for children and parents of a specific religion: Catholic, Jewish, and so on. Private agencies usually have more funding than do public agencies and thus are able to offer more in the way of counseling services to both biological and adoptive parents. The fees you will be asked to pay are usually somewhat higher at private than at public agencies. However, most agencies do have sliding fee scales based on a percentage of your yearly income.

The first thing you need to do is to find out which agencies are located in your area. Consult your telephone directory under "Adoption Agency," also call or write to your city, county, or state department of social services for information. Adoptive parents' groups in your area are another potential source of information, both to help you find out about specific agencies and also to provide you with information about which agencies are taking applications, what different agencies are looking for, what kinds of children each has available, and how best to present yourself to maximize your chances of being placed on their waiting list.

Information about how to locate adoptive parents' groups in your area may be obtained by contacting local agencies or through adoption information services such as the Open Door Society, the North American Council on Adoptable Children, the National Adoption Information Clearinghouse, and the newsletter OURS, of the organization Adoptive Families of America (see Adoption Resources).

In your search for an agency keep in mind that policies and practices of agencies differ widely. In making an initial selection you will want to determine whether or not the agency will consider applicants from your geographic area. Most of them require that you live within a certain distance in order to facilitate home study interviews and court appearances. In addition, you will want to determine if they accept applicants of your religious affiliation and if they place children in the age range you prefer.

The Application Procedure

The first hurdle that you have to master is finding an agency that will put you on their waiting list. Call or write whichever agencies you think may be receptive to you, informing them of your interest. Inquire whether the agency is accepting applications, if they handle children of the age you desire, whether you would be eligible to apply. Most agencies will not accept applications from couples wishing to adopt an infant if they do not have a fertility problem. Similarly, you may find that an agency may require that prospective parents be between given upper and lower age limits or that they have a requirement that you have been married at least two years before applying. You may also ask about special adoption services for older, minority, and special-needs children, and whether you would be considered for this type of placement. Some agencies will accept applications from couples who know they are fertile or from single individuals only if the applicant is willing to consider taking such a hard-to-place child.

If an agency is not taking applications, ask when they expect to be taking them again. Also ask for information regarding other agencies in your area that are currently accepting applications. They may also be able to tell you which agencies accept applications from fertile couples and single individuals.

Once you have found an agency that is accepting applications, you are ready to embark on the application process. The first step is to meet with the agency individually or with a group of applicants, depending on the policy of the given agency. This initial "information meeting" will be one that the agency uses to acquaint you with their policies and procedures. They will tell you what kinds of children they have available, what kinds of homes they are seeking, and what the anticipated waiting period is. They will also discuss the application process, agency requirements, and fees. You will be given an application form at the close of the meeting if you wish to pursue the application process further.

You will take the application form home with you, and when you have completed it, return it to the agency. Each agency has its own form. However, what is common to all of them is that they provide the agency with an effective screening device. This means that how you deal with this initial application may have a direct bearing on whether or not they will go on to approve you as an adoptive parent. As part of the application you will be asked to provide copies of some standard documents such as birth certificates, your marriage certificate, a divorce decree if either of you has been married and divorced in the past, proof of nationality, a W-2 tax form from the previous year, bank statements, insurance policies, and titles to any real estate that you may own. In addition, you will be asked to supply the agency with basic factual information about both you and your spouse. Some agencies request that each of you also submit an autobiography. It is customer for the agency to ask you to give them several references (somewhere between three and six, depending on the agency). References from your employer, your physician, or your clergyman may also be requested. A medical assessment of both your physical and emotional fitness, as well as your fertility status, will be requested from your physician. You will also be asked to fill out a financial report.

In filling out this application, you will naturally want to present yourselves in the most favorable light possible, in order to maximize your chances of obtaining the child you want. In her informative book *Beating the Adoption Game*, Cynthia Martin, a clinical psychologist with wide experience in all areas of adoption, presents many ideas about how to do this effectively. She advises that since the agency has what you want most, a child, either you tell them what they want to hear or you risk being turned down for not meeting their unstated criteria. For instance, your autobiography should emphasize your strengths, talents, and achievements, as well as those qualities and experiences that will demonstrate to the agency that you have what it takes to be a successful adoptive parent.

Similarly, it is critical that you select as references people who know and like you, and who can vouch for your fitness to raise a child. Before submitting names to the agency it will be worth your while to ask each potential reference whether they feel that they can write a strong letter on your behalf. Remember, this is a highly competitive arena, and a lukewarm letter may put you out of the running.

It is also advisable to be open-minded from the outset. For example, if you state that you want only a healthy white infant, and find the idea of adopting any other type of child unacceptable, some agencies will not even consider taking your application. Since there are few healthy white infants to be placed, agencies want to accept potential parents who are willing to consider adopting children from a wider spectrum. So, in order even to be in the running you might indicate that you are more flexible than you may actually be. Once your application has been accepted, and then approved, you still have the right to turn down any particular child who may be offered to you. Agreeing to consider a range of possibilities makes

you eligible to participate in the agency process; it does not obligate
you to accept a child you do not want.

The Home Study

Once you have returned your application form to the agency, you
will be assigned a social worker, who as a representative of the agency
will be the one to conduct an "adoption" or "home" study. Its purpose is to allow the agency to know you well enough so that they can
assess whether, in their opinion, you will be able to meet the needs of
the child they place with you. In addition, the home study attempts
to help you explore your thoughts and feelings about adoption, as
well as your feelings about being an adoptive parent. If you decide
that you want to continue to pursue adoption, your worker will use
the home study to help prepare you for the adjustments of adoption.
A fairly typical home study might consist of three interviews, two
conducted at the agency and a third at your home. In addition to
these joint interviews with you and your spouse, some agencies also
conduct separate interviews with each potential parent.

Although all agencies admit that it is difficult to predict who will
and who will not be a successful adoptive parent, each has its own
selection criteria. Trying to learn what an agency might look for in
prospective adoptive parents, we talked to an adoption worker who
has been employed by a private agency for many years. The following is a list of the kinds of attributes that this worker looks for.

1. Emotional Maturity — for example, how well each of you copes
with difficulty, uncertainty, and frustration and how you have dealt
with life crises.

2. Quality of Relationships with Others — how you relate to others;
whether you are able to accept differences in others; whether you
have the capacity to adjust and change in your relationships; and if
you are capable of warm and loving relationships.

3. Quality of the Marital Relationship — is your marriage stable? Do
you and your spouse treat each other with warmth and mutual
respect?

4. Feelings toward Children — how much experience have you had
with children? What kind of child do you desire, and why? Do you
and your spouse each — independently — desire a child?

5. *Flexibility* — this includes both how flexible you are able to be regarding the type of child you are willing to consider and whether you will be able to be an open and flexible parent.

6. *Acceptance of Infertility* — have you and your spouse come to terms with your inability to produce a biological child? Do you see adoption as an acceptable alternative way to have a child in your life?

7. *Readiness to Adopt* — are you aware of the implications of adoption for both you and your child? Are you able to accept the fact that your child will grow up with an extra parent (or two) always in the background, even if never present? Are you prepared to handle the issue of adoption with your child? Are you ready for parenthood? Is the marriage ready for children?

8. *Ability to Integrate a Child into Your Family* — if you already have biological children, will you be able to love an adopted child as much; will you be able to make him or her part of your family?

9. *Single Parenthood* — if you are single, are you able to support a child of your own? Can you provide a home for a child? Can you provide a child with a full life, including relationships with men, women, and families? Will a child be an addition to your life, and not a replacement for anything that is missing from it?

10. *Health Status* — are you physically and emotionally fit to raise a child? Do you have any condition that may interfere with your ability to be a parent, or that might shorten your life? (Most agencies claim that they have no absolute rules as to health requirements for adoptive parents — that each case is reviewed individually.)

11. *Financial Stability* — is your income adequate to raise a child? (Here, agencies claim to look, not at how much money you make, but rather, how well you manage your financial resources.) Many states are able to provide adoption subsidies. These are awarded primarily to low-income families and to foster parents who wish to adopt. In addition, most states offer both direct and medical subsidies to parents who adopt children with special needs.

After your home study is completed, your worker will submit the information she has collected to the agency for final consideration. Occasionally prospective adopters are rejected at this point. Some of the reasons that agencies give for rejecting applicants include the presence of marital problems, major medical problems, or personality problems in either parent.

If you are rejected, it is theoretically possible to reapply at a later time; the rejection is not irreversible. Find out why you were rejected. If your caseworker is unwilling to supply you with this information, demand of the agency administration that you be informed. Some couples have enlisted the aid of government officials in their local area, when they were unable to obtain an explanation by other means. Do what you have to in order to find out what you want to know. Once you learn the reason for being turned down, you will want to consider whether there is anything that you can do to reverse the decision. Remember, a rejection does not mean that you are bad or unfit: what it indicates is that you did not meet the agency's criteria for ideal adoptive parents.

Most likely, your application will be approved and you will be placed on the agency's waiting list for a child. As stated earlier, the length of time you will have to wait before a child is placed with you cannot be predicted. A wait of five to seven years is about average at the present time for a healthy infant, while the wait for a hard-to-place child will usually be far shorter than this.

After a long or short wait you will enter the pool of applicants that the agency is actively considering. When the agency locates a child that they feel will be suitable for you, your social worker will let you know that there is a child for you to consider. She will share with you information about the child's age, his general appearance, his race and national background, the history of his mother's pregnancy if he is newborn, his medical status, and, if the child is older, his personality traits. You will also be given some information about the child's biological parents: their age, race, religion, physical health, mental health, educational or work background, and information about why they are giving the child up for adoption. If after you learn about the child you are interested in considering him or her, the agency will arrange for you to meet him or her. When placing an older child, the agency usually holds several meetings before final placement is made. This gives both the adoptive parents and the child a chance to see if the placement is acceptable. Sometimes, a trial placement may be suggested.

Placement of the child in your home is usually followed by several more visits by the adoption worker. She will use these to assess how well everyone is adjusting, and to make a final assessment of the appropriateness of the placement. Although the child is in your home, he is not legally your child until the adoption is completed in court. How long after placement you will have to wait to go to court depends on the law in the state in which you live. The required waiting period is not just a pro forma requirement: although agencies rarely reclaim the children they place, they do have a legal right to do so.

In the case of a child older than twelve years, his consent will be required at the court hearing. This is the final step in making your long-awaited child truly yours.

INDEPENDENT, DIRECT, OR PRIVATE ADOPTION

Private adoption (the terms "independent' and "direct" adoption are synonymous with private adoption) and agency adoption can be pursued simultaneously. Therefore, unless a couple has a strong need to meet or know the biological mother (and/or father) of their adoptive child, or an unusually strong aversion to bureaucratic red tape, they can lose nothing by signing up with local agencies.

For couples that are unable to qualify with their local agencies, private adoption is an alternative means to adopting a child. If you do not qualify, it is very important that this setback not be blown out of proportion. Not qualifying does not in any way mean that you are unfit or incapable of being excellent parents. Rather, it is a reflection of the relative shortage of children available to the particular agency for placement.

In a private adoption the biological parents "place" their child with the adoptive parents "directly," or "independently" of agencies; in an agency adoption, the parents "place" a child with an agency, which, after obtaining custody, then "places" the child with a chosen couple.

In a private adoption, the burden of finding a child who is available for adoption falls on you rather than on a third party.

Private adoption is legal in all but the following states: Connecticut, Delaware, Massachusetts, Michigan, Minnesota, and North Dakota.

In some of these states agencies may be permitted to "facilitate" private placements through a process known as "identified adoption." There, a couple that knows of a baby available for a potential private placement can come within the law by hiring a licensed adoption agency to perform its usual function with respect to obtaining relinquishments and doing a home study, but treating the placement as a fait accompli.

It is important to find out what the specific legal process for private adoption is in your state. For example, Pennsylvania allows private adoption but requires a home study by a licensed social worker. The best source of information on this is likely to be a lawyer who specializes in adoption. Because adoption is not an everyday case for most lawyers, it is best to consult a lawyer who can speak from experience. Couples who have previously adopted a child through private adoption are a particularly good referral source. So too, are other lawyers, doctors, and social workers.

The procedures in private adoption vary greatly because they were created by state law. However, the general concept of private adoption is fairly uniform. Typically, a mother or mother-to-be reaches a decision that she does not have the ability or desire to raise her child. She concludes that adoption will best serve the child's interest, and learns of a couple that is willing and able to provide the child with parents and a loving, stable, permanent home. As soon as possible after birth, the child is physically placed with the adoptive parents, who then petition the court for an adoption decree that will legally create a parent-child relationship between them. After a period of some months (the exact waiting period differs from state to state), and with the benefit of a social service report (prepared by a government social agency) on the family, a judge terminates the biological parent-child relationship and grants the adoption.

In private adoption the final relinquishment papers are not signed until several months after the child is placed in the adoptive home, unlike agency adoption, where the mother has signed away her rights before placement. In a private adoption, then, since the adoption is not legally complete until several months after the child has been placed, the child could be reclaimed by the biological parents if they so wish. While this rarely occurs, it is a possibility and constitutes the single major drawback to private adoption: should the biological parents change their minds, the adoptive parents may have to give the child back. Since the regulations are subject to variations in state law, the applicable rules should be *thoroughly discussed* at the initial legal consultation. The prospect of having to return your child to its biological parents is frightening. It is an excellent reason for doing your best to evaluate the biological parents' certainty *before* the child is placed. Fortunately, "reclamations" or "reversals" are not very common. Although accurate statistics are hard to find, knowledgeable persons working in the adoption field have offered estimates of anywhere from 1 out of 25 to less than 1 in 50. If these figures are even remotely accurate, one's chances of losing a child because of parental change of heart are far less than of losing one during pregnancy. This somewhat grim reality is mentioned, however, as a reminder that getting a child, by whatever method, is risky.

Another aspect of private adoption which often worries prospective adoptive parents is that in private adoption the biological mother and father (if he is known) and the adoptive couple may know each other's identities. In practice, the amount of contact between biological and adoptive parents varies greatly. If all parties desire, they may get to know each other reasonably well. Alternatively, a mutual decision may be made to keep contact to a minimum. In the latter situation, a third party, a friend, doctor, lawyer, relative, or other intermediary, may assist the biological mother in finding out what she needs to know about the prospective adoptive parents.

Most couples find the lack of anonymity sometimes involved in private adoption disturbing at first. The usual fear is that, some day in the future, the biological mother will show up in their home or in the schoolyard and create an indescribably painful scene. Our experience has been that this is not the case. In fact, in sharp contrast to everyone's worst fears, meetings between the adoptive and biological parents are almost always very positive experiences. Seeing each other in the flesh can be extremely reassuring to all concerned. The biological parents can see for themselves that the adoptive parents are willing and able to love and care for their child. Similarly, a first-hand meeting gives the prospective adoptive parents an opportunity to evaluate in person how certain the biological parents are about their decision to give their child up for adoption. Usually, the reasons for relinquishing the child make sense, and it becomes obvious that fears of future harassment were largely fanciful.

Where such direct encounters between natural and adoptive parents do occur, they serve an additional function: the adoptive couple will be better able to satisfy the child's curiosity about his or her birth parents when the time comes to discuss the "facts of life."

Cost

Rumor has it that only wealthy couples, willing to buy a child, can engage in private adoption. In fact, although both birth-related expenses and legal fees for the adoption are customarily paid by the adoptive couple, it is illegal for anyone to profit unduly from the placement of a child. Black-market adoption, or baby selling, is not legal in any state.

Before you go ahead with a private adoption it is, however, important to know that, in general, the money you will pay out is nonrefundable. This means that in the event of a change of heart by the natural parents, they have no legal obligation to reimburse you. The reason for this is that the law requires that the parental consent be completely free and voluntary. An adoptive *placement* (before the final court appearance) is not a contractual relationship. It is viewed as an *offer* of a home by the prospective adoptive parents, who knowingly accept the risk involved.

The one way to be sure that costs are legitimate is to make certain that each expense is itemized and documented. Most couples have little difficulty finding out the going rate for a particular expense, and so are able to avoid being victimized. Only customary, reasonable fees can be charged.

It usually possible to get a fairly accurate idea about how much the adoption will cost before you decide to go through with it. Costs can vary from as low as $7,000 to as much as $20,000 or more. Of course, sometimes unplanned-for expenses do arise, such as uninsured medical bills that may be higher than anticipated (if, for example, a cesarean delivery must be performed), or if there are travel expenses for the mother or mother-to-be to deliver the child to you or for you to pick up the child from her.

Finding a Child to Adopt

How do you go about finding a child to adopt? There is no single answer to this question. Basically, what is necessary is to make contact, no matter how indirectly at first, with a woman who has a child she wishes to place. There are many different ways to accomplish this. Some people work through their doctor, lawyer, or clergyman. Others tell everyone they know that they are looking for a child, in the hope that a wide net will increase their chance of being successful. Generally, it is wise to let as many people as you can know that you are seeking a child to adopt. In addition, you might encourage your contacts to spread the word to everyone that they know. This is one time when you want the human gossip network to work for you. For example, you tell a friend who is a nurse. She tells all her friends and acquaintances, many of whom are also nurses, and so on. Remember, the more people out there who are looking for you, the better your chance of success.

Some people do not confine their search to their own circle of acquaintances or even to their own geographic area. Some write to people they know of all over the country. Blind mailings to obstetricians, family physicians, attorneys, clergymen, and "right-to-life" groups have been known to produce good leads. In states where it is legal to advertise, notices in city, suburban, rural, and college newspapers may turn up leads: ads put up in Laundromats, on church bulletin boards, or in grocery stores have also been successful. Your search can extend as far as the limits of your creativity, your energy, or your financial resources — it all depends on how determined you are.

Since it is impossible to predict where and when a lead will appear, it is necessary that you prepare yourself for instant success before you let the word out. Paul and Joan had this experience. Two weeks after writing a letter to their physician uncle in another state, they received a call from a colleague of his. He informed them that he had a patient who had just delivered a healthy boy and was looking for a couple to adopt the child. After some frantic searching they were able to locate a lawyer who was knowledgeable about private adoption in their state. With the help of their newly found lawyer they were able within a week's time to evaluate the lead that had come their way, follow it up, and arrange for the adoption of their son.

Of course, not everyone is as fortunate as Paul and Joan. Sometimes it takes a lot more searching before a lead is unearthed. Sometimes one that at first looked promising does not work out. It cannot be overemphasized that once a possibility is located it must be carefully evaluated; some are better than others. Before committing yourself emotionally or financially, you should obtain as much information as possible. Areas that are important to find out about include the certainty of the birth parents' decision to relinquish the child, the parents' health, and if the child is already born, his or her health, estimated costs, and any potential legal problems that may exist.

It is important that you feel good about a lead before getting too deeply involved. Acting out of a sense of desperation is a greater mistake than being too choosy. There will be other possibilities, and it is a bad idea to go against one's better judgment.

It is also a good idea to be ready for something to go wrong. Leads have been known to fizzle before a placement occurs. The decision to relinquish one's child is a difficult one for most people. Not infrequently, especially around the time of the birth, there is a change of heart by the biological parent or parents. The couple that holds back emotionally until the actual placement occurs is best able to cope with these "adoptive miscarriages" and to get ready for the next possibility.

The Placement

Assuming all goes well, the actual placement usually takes place as soon as possible. With newborns, if the biological parent agrees, the adoptive couple can even take care of the baby in the nursery. At the birth parents' option and when state law permits, they can sign the child out of the hospital to the adoptive parents or make the transfer personally outside.

Once the child is placed in the adoptive home, the legal petition for adoption is filed. Thereafter, a state social agency does an investigation and makes a report, which is filed with the court. The report usually contains a recommendation that the adoption be granted and gives background information. The information, which was gathered by the adoption worker, usually includes biographical facts about the adoptive couple and biological parents, medical information, references, and other relevant data.

Finally, when the report has been filed, the consents of the biological parents have been taken, and the statutory time period of waiting (if any) has gone by, the adoption is completed in court.

The court appearance is usually only a formality and lasts only a few minutes. Judges tend to give solemn advice or make friendly jokes before sending the happy parents on their way. One couple was told by the judge, "I adopted a child myself. We figured we needed some brains and good looks in the family."

INTERCOUNTRY ADOPTION

In an intercountry, or international, adoption, you, the adoptive parent, adopt a child born in another country. The adoption is legalized either in the country of the child's birth or in your state of residence in the United States (depending on various factors, including your state's laws and the laws of the particular foreign country).

Is Intercountry Adoption a Possibility for You?

If you've made the decision to adopt a child, if you have positive feelings about becoming a transracial/transcultural family forever, if you can accept the unknowns in the life of a foreign-born child, if you have the patience, energy, flexibility, and determination to deal with the complexities of intercountry adoption, if you have the financial resources to meet the costs of intercountry adoption — then intercountry adoption could be an option for you in building a family through adoption.

In educating yourself about intercountry adoption, you'll find out about the need for racial and cultural awareness if your family is to become transracial and transcultural. You'll read and hear about the benefits of learning about your child's heritage — about racial and cultural origins — and about teaching the whole family as your child grows. It's an exciting and stimulating process.

Who Chooses Intercountry Adoption?

People who choose intercountry adoption are often couples who would qualify for domestic agency adoption of a healthy infant but who don't want to wait five years or longer, couples (or single persons) who are rejected by local agencies for domestic infant adoption for a variety of reasons (for example, their age or having two or more children at home already — even if these are children from a previous marriage — or being single), and people who actively seek to adopt foreign-born special-needs children: school-age children, sibling groups, physically and/or mentally challenged children.

The Children

The children available for international adoption come from countries with widespread poverty, countries perhaps suffering the turmoil of war or natural disasters, countries that cannot, at present, provide for their homeless children, countries that look favorably on placing children for adoption internationally, countries where adoption is not an accepted cultural practice, where biological family ties are intensely strong, where an impoverished family cannot feed all of its children, where the unwed mother and the illegitimate child are social outcasts, where there is no bright future for the abandoned or orphaned child — where if the child indeed survives infancy and early childhood, he may grow up in an orphanage, in a hospital, in a prison, or simply in the streets.

In 1991, United States citizens were adopting children almost exclusively from Latin America (Colombia, Guatemala, Honduras, Peru, Paraguay, Bolivia, and Chile), from Eastern Europe (Romania, Bulgaria, and the Soviet Union) and from Asia (the Philippines, India, and a small number from Korea). In some of these countries, there are many children who can be legally freed for adoption, and the process of international adoption is straightforward and fairly routine; in other countries, there are very few children actually available for international adoption and the procedures may be quite complicated and/or time-consuming.

Babies are usually available through international adoption agencies as well as through private contacts. At times, your wait for an infant could be much longer (many months, even two years or longer) than the wait for a preschool or school-age child, a sibling group, or a handicapped child. At other times, the offer of an infant might come within a few months after you've been accepted by your foreign contact or by the United States–based agency helping you with your adoption.

As part of the home study and application process, you'll consider the age range that you'd be able to accept, being as flexible as possible, yet honest about your feelings. Be aware, too, that babies and older children with correctable medical problems (cleft palate, for instance) are often considered hard to place and are therefore readily available for adoption.

Where Do You Start?

"Put as many irons in the fire as you can" : . . . valuable advice for prospective adoptive parents who are pursuing *any* kind of adoption. What exactly does this mean for you if you are interested in intercountry adoption? First, it's always helpful to tell as many people as you can that you are planning to adopt and that you are interested in intercountry adoption. This increases your chances of (1) hearing about new developments: for example, new agencies, new sources of children; (2) being given personal contacts in foreign countries; (3) learning about individual families and/or adoptive parents' groups in your area who've had experience in intercountry adoption and would gladly share knowledge and give you the opportunity to meet their children.

You might begin cautiously by attending an information meeting offered by an adoption agency or an adoptive parents' group; by reading materials on intercountry adoption, transracial adoption, and the countries involved in intercountry adoption; by talking to people who've adopted internationally and meeting their children. You might even find a course for prospective adoptive parents taught at a local college. NOTE: It doesn't hurt — and costs so little — to do all these things at once even as you develop your thoughts about adopting, confirm your desires, and gather information on *all* possible sources for a child.

The best place to start is with a adoptive parents' support group that has members who are knowledgeable about intercountry adoptions. Your contact can acquaint you with state and federal regulations affecting intercountry adoption; with the countries most likely to be placing children for international adoption with United States citizens; with your local sources (agency or private social worker) for a home study (federal law requires a home study for all inter-country adoptions). The parents' group can also give you up-to-date information about United States–based international adoption agencies and possibly about foreign contacts for parent-initiated adoptions.

Types of Intercountry Adoption

There are two types of intercountry adoption: agency (agency-to-agency) adoptions and parent-initiated adoptions. In the former, a United States adoption agency has made child-placing agreements with a foreign agency or with a United States–based international adoption agency. For the prospective adoptive parents, most of the paperwork involved in this process is taken care of by the agencies. After your applications have been accepted and your home study has been approved, a child is selected and offered to you (all of these steps involve time and [im]patient waiting!). You can expect to receive a photograph of the child you are considering as well as his or her medical and social histories. Often, once a placement is made, the child is escorted to the United States, though sometimes parents must travel to the child's country in order to bring him or her home.

In parent-initiated adoptions, the prospective adoptive parents must, for the most part, arrange the adoption themselves: that is, you as the adopter find the foreign source willing to accept your application for a child; you obtain a home study; you are personally responsible for sending official translations of all documents to the proper authorities of the country where you're planning to adopt; you communicate directly with your foreign contact (keeping the local social worker informed) and with the foreign attorney; you work directly with the United States Immigration Service to obtain an entry visa for your child; and you travel to your child's country to escort the child home.

The language barrier and the lack of personal or face-to-face contact with your source may pose risks or present complications that are usually avoidable with agency adoptions. On the other hand, some people view these factors merely as a challenge.

Costs

Intercountry adoption is not an inexpensive way to adopt a child. Costs range from $10,000 to $15,000, depending on the country. Fees you should expect to pay in any intercountry adoption are your local home study fee (these vary greatly), an immigration fee for your child's visa, and air fare for you and/or your child. In addition, you may pay a fee to the foreign agency placing your child; a fee to a liaison agency helping in the placement; translation fees; notarization, verification, and authentication fees. You may want to make a donation to the organization that cared for your child before the adoption (an orphanage, for example), and you may want to send or take supplies needed in caring for infants and children.

Advice from Those Who Chose Intercountry Adoption: The Process Is Often Hard Work, but the Results Are Worth It!

It's important to bear in mind that the adoption picture could change at any time in a particular country (and that new state or federal laws enacted in the United States *or* new interpretations of existing regulations could affect your intercountry adoption as well). For example, political unrest and a change of government can dramatically and suddenly alter the adoption situation. This is where your ability to be flexible and patient is essential.

Realize that you'll need fortitude, patience, optimism, and determination in pursuing intercountry adoption. For an agency-assisted intercountry adoption, you'll probably needs lots of patience and fortitude; for a parent-initiated intercountry adoption, you'll need a great deal of energy and determination. You'll *always* need optimism — and that can be bolstered by seeking the reassuring support of other adoptive parents and by reading everything you can in the adoption literature. Of course, your determination and creative energy in pursuing intercountry adoption will still be the key to finding your child.

Acknowledgments

Surviving Pregnancy Loss is the product of many people's efforts. We are grateful to all who talked with us, filled out our lengthy questionnaire, shared their experiences, and often, despite their own pain, helped and encouraged us along the way.

Special thanks to the following people for contributing a detailed account of their personal experiences: Craig Anderson for "The Husband's Experience"; Judith Wrubel for "Ectopic Pregnancy: One Woman's Experience"; Margaret S. Ross, M.D., for "Miscarriage: One Woman's Experience"; Charlene Arcidiacono for "Stillbirth: One Woman's Experience"; and Kate Thompson for "Assisted Reproductive Technology: One Woman's Experience." We are indebted to each of you for sharing so much, your hopes and fears, your pain and disappointment, your words of advice and your spirit to survive.

Our warm thanks also to the friends and colleagues whose generous contributions we warmly appreciate: Tate Snyder for "Intercountry Adoption"; Darlene Peck, R.N., for sharing her work on the role of the health care professional; Sal Lopes for sharing his thoughts about how men experience the loss of a pregnancy; Lora Tessman, Ph.D., Lois Eichler, Ph.D., and Miriam Mazor, M.D., for many germinative conversations; Karen Cohen for coleading the original miscarriage support group and for collaborating on subsequent projects; Robert H. Friedman, M.D., for his help and support throughout; Marc Gradstein, attorney-at-law, for serving as consultant on legal issues and for his contribution to the private adoption chapter; Mary Tondorf-Dick, our thoughtful and sensitive editor, who shared our vision and helped it take form.

Thanks also go to Bette Greene, Alaina Anderson, Lee Dauber, Lauren Tofias, Hannah Hecht, Stephanie Blumberg, Cecile Terrien Lampton and David Lampton, Susan Laughlin, D.S.W., Alexis Aquino Mackles, Annelise Rothman, Linda Ataide, R.N., Donna

Benedict, R.N., Jane Butler, R.N., Joan M. Oustifine, R.N., Lowell
Cooper, Ph.D., Philip J. Hoffman, M.D., Russell K. Laros, M.D.,
Lawrence Mackles, M.D., Peter McConarty, M.D., David S. Chapin,
M.D., Annie Liau, M.D., and David Hagen, M.D.

We would like to thank The Compassionate Friends, Resolve,
Inc., and Sister Jane Marie Lamb, SHARE Chairperson, for assist-
ing us in collecting the information about support organizations,
and we are grateful to Barbara Thayer, M.S., and Wayne Miller,
M.D., of Prenatal Diagnostic Center, Inc., for sharing their vast
experience with us.

We also would like to thank Kathy Gossett, Eileen Cox, Jordana
Friedman, Sharon Pellegrino, and Julie S. Roberts for their help
with the manuscript. A special thanks to Kathleen Kendrick for her
invaluable contribution and to Myra Green for all her help.

We are deeply indebted to Robert Glass, M.D., who offered continual encouragement and advice throughout the writing of this
book, generously gave of his time to write a foreword, shared his
expertise on the medical aspects of pregnancy loss, and served as a
sounding board through the years of researching and writing.

Appendix: Resources

National Organizations

Alliance of Genetic Support Groups
Suite 800
1001 22nd Street, N.W.
Washington, D.C. 20037
(800) 336-GENE

AMEND (Aiding a Mother Experiencing Neonatal Death)
National Headquarters
Mrs. Maureen Connelly
4324 Berrywick Terrace
St. Louis, MO 63128
(314) 487-7582

American Fertility Society
Joyce Zeitz
2140 11th Avenue South
Suite 200
Birmingham, AL 35205-2800
(205) 933-8494

Beyond Prenatal Choice
Genetics Department, CHNMC
111 Michigan Avenue, N.W.
Washington, D.C. 20010

The Compassionate Friends
P.O. Box 3696
Oak Brook, IL 60522-3696
(708) 990-0010

Cystic Fibrosis Foundation
6931 Arlington Road
Bethesda, MD 20184
(800) FIGHT-CF

Dalkon Shield Information Network
Karen Hicks
626 Center Street
Bethlehem, PA 18018
(215) 867-6577

Endometriosis Association
International Headquarters
8585 North 76th Place
Milwaukee, WI 53223
(800) 992-3636

HAND (Help After Neonatal Death)
P.O. Box 62
San Anselmo, CA 94960
(415) 492-0720

Huntington's Disease Society of America
140 W. 22nd Street
New York, NY 10010
(800) 345-HDSA

March of Dimes Birth Defects Foundation
1275 Mamaroneck Avenue
White Plains, NY 10605
(914) 428-7100

National Clearinghouse for Human Genetic Diseases
1776 East Jefferson Street
Rockville, MD 20852

National Down Syndrome Congress
1800 Dempster
Park Ridge, IL 60068-1146
(800) 232-6372

National Hemophilia Foundation
Soho Building
110 Green Street
New York, NY 10012
(212) 219-8180

National Society of Genetic Counselors
233 Canterbury Drive
Wallingford, PA 19086
(215) 872-7608

*National Sudden Infant Death Syndrome
   Foundation*
Two Metro Plaza
Suite 205
8240 Professional Place
Landover, MD 20785

*National Tay Sachs and Allied Diseases
   Association*
2001 Beacon Street
Suite 304
Brookline, MA 02146
(617) 277-4463

Resolve, Inc.
Ann Petter, Executive Director
P.O. Box 474
Belmont, MA 02178
(617) 643-2424

*SHARE (A Source of Help in Airing
   and Resolving Experiences)*
National Headquarters
St. John's Hospital
800 East Carpenter Street
Springfield, IL 62702
(217) 544-6464

Spina Bifida Association of America
1700 Rockville Pike
Suite 250
Rockville, MD 20852

State-by-State Organizations

ALABAMA

AMI Brookwood Medical Center
John Gregory and Cynthia Bullard
2010 Brookwood Medical Center
    Drive
Birmingham 35209
(205) 877-1936/5389

ALASKA

Parents Reaching Out
Lisa Fleisher
P.O. Box 14-2874
Anchorage 99514
(907) 333-2935

SHARE
Elizabeth McWilliams
P.O. Box 14-2874
Anchorage 99514

OUR Newsletter
Jean Kollantai
P.O. Box 1064
Palmer 99645
(907) 745-2706

Parents Reaching Out
Palmer
(907) 745-2706

Parents Reaching Out
Wasilla
(907) 745-1632

ARIZONA

Compassionate Friends / Infant Group
Cindy Chambers
3221 E. Campobello Drive
Phoenix 85032
(602) 971-6018

SHARE
Palo Verde Hospital
P.O. Box 41208
Tucson 85717
(602) 322-4340

ARKANSAS

AMEND of Northwest Arkansas
Sandra Hopkins
1680 E. Shadowridge Drive
Fayetteville 72701
(501) 521-1860

Resolve Through Sharing
Sylvia Tharp
Quachita Memorial Hospital
Olive at Broadway Street, Box
    1137
Hot Springs 71901
(501) 624-5702

AMEND
Box 7062
Jonesboro 72403

*SHARE/University of Arkansas Medical
    Science*
Cindy Westcott
4301 West Markham Slot #518
Little Rock 72205
(501) 661-5000

CALIFORNIA

Sharing Parents of Kern County
Twenty-four-Hour Hot Line
4909 Stockdale Highway,
    Box 333
Bakersfield 93309
(805) 366-6323

SAND (Support After Neonatal Death)
Janet Kirksey
3001 Colby Street
Berkeley 94725
(415) 540-1571

HOPING (Helping Other Parents In
    Natural Grief)
8200 Owensmouth Avenue #14
Canoga Park 91304

SAIL (Support After Infant &
    Pregnancy Loss)
Eden Hospital/Social Services
    Department
20103 Lake Chabot Road
Castro Valley 94579
(415) 537-1234, Extension 5043

Respond — Chico
Kathy Sorrels
10 Forest Creek Avenue
Chico 95926

SHARE
Diane Bremseth
436 Loverne Avenue
Clovis 93612
(209) 299-0008

HOPING of Colton/San Bernardino
Marilyn Noordhof
752 Plumwood Street
Colton 92324
(714) 825-2469

Empty Arms
Lori Lingenfelter
8773 Comet Street
Cucumonga 91730
(714) 982-6074

HOPE (Helping Other Parents
    Endure) — Eureka
Debra Jones
911 Third Street
Eureka 95501

SHARE
Sister Ann Keating
1111 East Spruce, P.O. Box 27500
Fresno 93729
(209) 449-5222

HOPING of Orange County
Cherie Beckmeyer
11022 Flynn
Garden Grove 92640
(714) 635-4486

Parental Loss Group
Janice and David Phillips
222 South Russ Street
King City 93930
(407) 385-4457

Hoping & Sharing of Long Beach
Marie Teague
5335 Carita Street
Long Beach 90808
(213) 425-4889

Moment by Moment
Patsy Jones
Cedars-Sinai Medical Center
8700 Beverly Boulevard, Room 3506
Los Angeles 90048
(213) 855-5357

HAND of Santa Clara County
Pam Puetsch
P.O. Box 341
Los Gatos 95031
(408) 732-3228

SHARE
Sofia Close
3347 Courtland Avenue
Oakland 94619

Sharing Parents
Leslie Massey, RN
Marshall Hospital
Marshall Way
Placerville 95667
(916) 626-2679

PACS (Parents Adjusting through
    Caring)
Dianne Van Loon
YWCA
8172 Magnolia
Riverside 92504
(714) 688-5531

Sharing Parents
Sacramento
(916) 424-5150

HAND
Ginger Valen
P.O. Box 62
San Anselmo 94960

HAND of the Peninsula
Emily Corpos, Coordinator
257 Fir Street
San Carlos 94070
(415) 591-0283

Empty Cradle
April R. Fout
4869 Marlborough Drive
San Diego 92116
(619) 692-2144

HAND
P.O. Box 3805
San Francisco 94119

SAND
Niva Jones
Department of Social Services
3700 California
San Francisco 94118
(415) 387-8700

HAND
Anna Heffron
Apple Family Center
70 Skyview Terrace
San Rafael 94903
(415) 492-0720

Coping
Yvonne Fundingsland
561 Northview Road
Santa Barbara 93105
(805) 682-8020, 682-7529

Parents' Bereavement Outreach
Lee Schmidt, RN
535 16th Street
Santa Monica 90402
(213) 825-2450

Bereavement Parents & Mourning After
Santa Rosa Memorial Hospital
1165 Montgomery Drive
Santa Rosa 95402
(707) 546-3210

HAND of Santa Cruz
Lisa Jones
4382 Ranchero Drive
Soquel 95073
(408) 475-4188

SHARE
Emily Rivera
Keweah Delta Hospital
400 West Mineral King
Visalia 93291
(209) 625-2211

Grief Counseling
Susan Breed
P.O. Box 4652
Walnut Creek 94596
(415) 944-0645

COLORADO

Humana — SHARE
Kathy McGraw, Director
1501 South Potomac Street
Aurora 80012
(303) 695-2600

Stillborn/Newborn Loss Support Group
M. Lattanzi
Boulder County Hospice
2825 Marine Street
Boulder 80303
(303) 449-7740

Compassionate Friends
Lynn Berns
16 East Platte Avenue
Colorado Springs 80903
(719) 633-8888

HOPING
Joyce Boyles
11070 Hardy Road
Colorado Springs 80908

Rose Fetal & Newborn Loss Program
Dorotha Graham Cicchinelli or
  Barbara Todd
4567 East 9th Avenue, Parent
  Education Department
Denver 80220
(303) 320-2764, 320-2713

SHARE
Rhonda Welch
3512 Lilac Lane
Evans 80620
(303) 330-1629

HOPING of Larimer County
Lisa Rossi
Poudre Valley Hospital
Fort Collins 80524
(303) 484-4318

*Association for Recognizing Life of
  Stillborns*
11470 West Powers Avenue
Littleton 80127

HOPING
Kathy Morrissey
2445 Courtney Drive
Loveland 80537

North Area SHARE
Rita Beam, RN, and Nancy Sneath,
  MSW
Humana Hospital, Mount View, and
  Saint Anthony's
9191 Grant Street
Thornton 80229
(303) 450-4520

CONNECTICUT

SHARE
Robin Wheeler, RNC
227 Stadley Rough Road
Danbury 06811
(203) 744-4658

SHARE of Greater Bridgeport
Dolores De Rita
99 Birch Road
Fairfield 06430
(203) 255-8955

AID (Aid in Infant Death)
Saint Francis Hospital and Medical
  Center
114 Woodland Street
Hartford 06105
(203) 548-4000

Newborn Death Support Group
Women's Center of Southeastern
  Connecticut
Donna Goldman, MA
120 Broad Street
New London 06339
(203) 447-0366

SHARE
Roberta Kemp, RN, BSN, and Susan
  Lamay, RN
Sharon Hospital
Hospital Hill Road
Sharon 06069
(203) 364-4120 or -4124

SHARE of Greater Waterbury
Mary Beth Pratt or Carol Doiron
1960 Bucks Hill Road, Southbury
  06488, or 67 Harrison Lane,
  Bethlehem 06488
(203) 264-7644 or 266-5974

AID
Susan Braren
27 Anderson Road
Tolland 06084
(203) 872-0326

Uphold
Mary Lou Greer
100 Teeter Rock Road
Trumbull 06611
(203) 377-2056

SHARE
Mary Hanka/Lisa Brown
48 Chestnut Street/65 Chestnut
  Street
Willimantic 06226
(203) 456-8101

HOPE
Nancy Walker
89 Maple View
Woodbridge 06525
(203) 397-5200

DELAWARE

Unite, Inc.
April Palekar, RN
Beebe Hospital
Lewes 19958

Loving Arms Parents' Support Group
Marie Hughes
Medical Center of Delaware
P.O. Box 6001
Newark 19718
(302) 733-2375

HOPING
Reverend Walters
Grace United Methodist Church
Wilmington 19801

Parents' Support Groups
Pat Ohrams
Delaware Medical Center
1902 Gheen Road
Wilmington 19808
(302) 994-9287

FLORIDA

Empty Arms
Nancy Brubaker
3505 65th Street West
Bradenton 33529
(813) 959-0323, 977-2090

HOPING
Jane Paul
3609 S.E. 5th Court
Cape Coral 33904
(813) 542-0270

Resolve Through Sharing
Morton Plant Hospital
OB/RN Maternal/Child Services
323 Jeffords Street
Clearwater 34616

Caring Friends
Dolores McCrory
Lake County, Star Route 3, Box 844
Eustis 32726
(904) 357-9876

HOPING
Evelyn Stetson
941 Adelphia Court
Fort Myers 33907
(813) 481-8173

Resolve Through Sharing
Sandra Mays
Memorial Medical Center
3625 University Boulevard South
Jacksonville 32216
(904) 399-6111

Resolve Through Sharing
Janie Zachary
Saint Vincent Medical Center
1800 Barrs Street, Box 2982
Jacksonville 32203
(904) 387-7300

SHARE — Leesburg, Florida
Judy Fischer
9848 Rosemary Lane
Leesburg 34788
(904) 728-5056, 589-3333

SHARE
Pat Stauber
North Shore Medical Center
1100 N.W. 95th Street
Miami 33150
(305) 835-6165

SHARE
Darlene Moon, RN
Baptist Hospital of Miami, Inc.
8900 North Kendall Drive
Miami 33176
(305) 596-1960, Extension 6658

Caring Friends
Jennifer Kunz
4809 Figwood Lane
Orlando 32808
(305) 293-1766

COPES
Pat Burt
232 Riverbeach
Ormond Beach 32074
(904) 677-4453

AMEND
Kim Petrie, Director
5241 Rowe Trail
Pace 32571
(904) 994-4368

*Neonatal & Early Infant Death Support
   Group*
Shelly Wortman
Center for Counseling Services
140 South University Avenue
Plantation 33324
(305) 475-1371

SHARE
Terry Johnson, ARNP, RNC
All Children's Hospital
801 Sixth Street South
St. Petersburg 33701
(813) 892-4264

AMEND
Karen M. Frazier
15405 Fenton Place
Tampa 33647
(813) 972-2273, 977-2090

Caring Friends
Margie White
Seminole County, 104 Moss Road
Winter Springs 32708
(305) 327-0347

GEORGIA

Preemie Parents' Support Group
Lisa Cohen
Northside Hospital
1000 Johnson Ferry Road, NE
Atlanta 30042
(404) 851-8000

SHARE
Larry M. Connolly
Piedmont Hospitals
1968 Peachtree Road, NW
Atlanta 30309
(404) 350-2222

HAWAII

HOPING
Judy Boomer
46-398 Holopu Place
Kaneohe 96744
(808) 834-5333

IDAHO

SHARE of Idaho
Nanci Dunbar
P.O. Box 1225
Boise 83701
(208) 342-7226

SHARE
Kellie Gonzalez
5370 Pinon Place
Mountain Home AFB 83648
(208) 832-7077

ILLINOIS

AMEND of Madison County
Jane Borman
2209 Gillis
Alton 62002
(618) 466-7129

Compassionate Friends
N.W. Suburban Chapter
800 W. Central Road
Arlington Heights 60005
(312) 259-1000

SHARE
Sister Jane Marie Lamb
St. Elizabeth's Hospital
211 S. Third Street
Belleville 62222
(618) 234-2120, 234-2415

SHARE
Elizabeth Johnson
409 W. Eighth
Belvidere 61008
(815) 544-4704

SHARE
Mrs. Debbie Drechney
St. Joseph's Hospital
437 Garden Drive
Belvidere 61008
(815) 544-0733

*Living With the Loss of a
   Child — Support Group*
Chaplain Judith Grimler
2200 East Washington
Bloomington 61701
(309) 662-3311

SHARE
Helen Essenpreis
St. Joseph's Hospital
Jamestown Road
Breese 62230
(618) 526-4511

SHARE of Rushville
Melissa Mathis
114 North Jackson Street
Browning 62624
(217) 322-4321

ILAC (I Lost A Child)
Elenie Smith, RNC
Memorial Hospital
404 West Main Street
Carbondale 62901
(618) 549-0721, Extension 5200

SHARE
Linda Whited, RN
718 Ashton Lane South
Champaign 61820
(217) 359-5480

Caring/Understanding Team
M. Heinz
Ravenwood Hospital Medical Center
4500 N. Winchester
Chicago 60640
(312) 878-4300

Coping Aid
Judy Friedrichs
1753 Congress Parkway
Chicago 60612
(312) 942-5068

Together in the Loss of a Child
Donna Stanislawski or Lynn Galuska
  Elsen
Northwestern Memorial Hospital
333 East Superior, Labor and
  Delivery Department
Chicago 60611
(312) 908-7600, 908-7680

TOUCH
Barbara Julion
Bethany Hospital
3435 W. Van Buren
Chicago 60624
(312) 638-6824

SHARE
Agnes Kolbeck, Pastoral Care
St. Mary's Hospital
1800 E. Lake Shore Drive
Decatur 62525
(217) 429-2966

Sauk Valley SHARE
Mary Kay Frey
403 E. 3rd Street
Dixon 61021
(815) 289-5531

SHARE
Tricia Horst
Quad Cities Group
618 33rd Avenue
East Moline 61244
(309) 755-1945

SHARE of Effingham
Deb Rubach
503 North Maple Street
Effingham 62401
(217) 347-1321

*Support Center for Perinatal/Childhood
  Death*
Laya Frischer
Evanston Hospital, 2WH
2650 Ridge Avenue
Evanston 60201
(708) 570-2882

Resolve Through Sharing
M. Kaufman, RN, W. Bingner, RN,
  and G. Hagemann
Freeport Memorial Hospital
1045 W. Stephenson Street
Freeport 61032
(815) 235-0244

SHARE
Sandra Fisk
Galesburg Cottage Hospital
695 N. Kellogg Street
Galesburg 61401
(309) 343-8131, Extension 210

West Suburban Compassionate Friends
Joanne and Greg Matzke
First Street and Park Avenue
Hinsdale 60521
(312) 455-6808, 323-2706

SHARE
Kathy Shank
Passavant Hospital
1600 W. Walnut Street
Jacksonville 62650
(217) 245-9541, Extension 184

SHARE
Marilyn James
Route 1
Jewett 62436
(217) 683-2210

SHARE
Cindy Waters
McDonough District Hospitals
525 E. Grant Street
Macomb 61455
(309) 833-4101

AMEND/ILAC
Malinda Sawyer
Route #5, Box 353
Marion 62959

Sharing Parents
Karen Kronk, RN
Anderson Hospital
Route 162, Route 159, P.O. Box
  1000
Maryville 62294
(618) 288-5711, Extension 466

SHARE
Hugh Smith
Sarah Bush Lincoln Health Center
P.O. Box 372, East Route 16
Mattoon 61938
(217) 258-2392

SHARE
Linda Bronersky
Loyola University Medical Center
2160 South First Avenue
Maywood 60153
(312) 531-4044, 531-3056

SHARE
Debbie Vrtis, Laura Malo
1709 Pleasant Avenue
McHenry 60050
(815) 344-0756, 338-2249

SHARE
Gregory and Joanne Matzke
10301 Medill
Melrose Park 60164

Combined Grief Support
Carol Hughey, RN
Good Samaritan Regional Health
  Center
605 N. 12th
Mt. Vernon 62864
(618) 242-4600, Extensions 5580,
  5540

Grieving Parents' Support Network
Cindy Scroggins
1419 Chadwick Drive
Normal 61716
(309) 454-7000

Compassionate Friends
National Office
P.O. Box 3696
Oak Brook 60522
(708) 990-0010

Caring Connection
Reverend Sherry Miller, Chaplain
Christ Hospital and Medical Center
4440 West 95th Street
Oak Lawn 60453
(708) 857-5175

Caretakers
Robert J. Long
West Suburban Hospital
Erie at Austin Boulevard
Oak Park 60302
(708) 386-8457

Richland Memorial Hospital
Kathy Bunting
800 East Locust
Olney 62450
(618) 395-2131

Coffee and Comfort
Mrs. Diane Wendt
7500 W. Sycamore Drive
Orland Park 60462
(708) 460-1392

Empty Arms
C. Basham
Community Hospital of Ottawa
1100 E. Norris Drive
Ottawa 61350
(815) 433-3100, 434-2152

HOLD (Healing Our Lost Dreams)
Chaplain Carol Stephens
Lutheran General Hospital
1775 Dempster Street
Park Ridge 60068
(312) 696-6395

Heart of Illinois SHARE
Billie Rocke
St. Francis Medical Center
530 N.E. Glen Oak Avenue
Peoria 61637
(309) 655-2090

Illinois SHARE
Clairann Nicklin
Methodist Medical Center
211 N.E. Glen Oak Avenue
Peoria 61636
(309) 672-4850, 686-5806

MIS
Lois Wahrenburg
2402 Lohman Road
Peoria 61604
(309) 674-0213, 685-5010

Empty Arms (A SHARE Group)
Nancy Pormenter
Illinois Community Hospital
925 West Street
Peru 61354
(815) 223-3300, Extension 443

SHARE of Quincy
Jan Webb, DVS
Blessing Hospital
Box C-3
Quincy 62305
(217) 223-5811, Extension 1405

SHARE Group
Kristi Tuescher, LSW, ACSW
2400 N. Rockton Avenue
Rockford 61103
(815) 968-6861

SHARE
Sister Jane Marie Lamb
St. John's Hospital
800 East Carpenter
Springfield 62702

SHARE
Judy Hinton, RN
Covenant Medical Center
1400 West Park
Urbana 61801
(217) 337-2226

SHARE
Joye Eyman
Route 1
Vandalia 62471
(618) 283-0425

PACES
Susan Gittings
P.O. Box 213
Western Springs 60558
(312) 848-1630

*Loyola Premature High Risk Infant
    Parents' Association*
1021 Garner
Wheaton 60187
(312) 852-1910

INDIANA

Jill Bowles
2920 V Street
Bedford 47421

Resolve Through Sharing
Michele K. Wood
St. Francis Hospital
1600 Albany Street
Beech Grove 46107
(317) 781-1281

SHARE
M. Risley
Bartholomew County Hospital
2400 East Seventeenth Street
Columbus 47201
(812) 379-4441

Bereaved Parents/Friends of Children
Linda Runden
717 North Capitol Avenue
Corydon 47112
(812) 738-3277

HOPE
Rita Walker, RN
Elkhart General Hospital
600 East Boulevard
Elkhart 46515
(219) 523-3275

SHARE
Mary Beteh Lodato, RNC, MSN
St. Mary's Medical Center
3700 Washington Avenue
Evansville 47711
(812) 867-0063

Tri-County SHARE
Susan Yingling
30 West 975 South
Fairmount 46928
(317) 948-5112

Project Comfort
Parkview Hospital
2200 Randalia Drive
Fort Wayne 46805
(219) 484-6636

Neo Fight
Pam Dickerson
4815 North Kenyon Drive
Indianapolis 46226

Resolve Through Sharing
Mary Nell Williams/Judy Marich
Saint Vincent Hospital and Health
   Care Center
2001 West 86th Street
Indianapolis 46260
(317) 871-2028

SHARE
Joan Callahan
Community Hospital
1500 North Ritter Avenue,
   Department 670
Indianapolis 46219
(317) 353-5505

SHARE Outreach
Sherry Hutchins
103 West Diamond Street
Kendallville 46755
(219) 347-3209 or 347-3826

SHARE
Julie Sims
659 N. 7th Street
Lafayette 47901
(317) 742-6574

SHARE
Pat Parr
305 N. Detroit Street
LaGrange 46761
(219) 463-7266

Mrs. William Bear
2329 Hargan Drive
Madison 47250

Parents Beginning Again
Vickie Johnson
Floyd Memorial Hospital
1850 State Street
New Albany 47150
(812) 948-7682

Compassionate Friends
Nancy Prange
2606 Pleasant
South Bend 46615
(219) 233-5915

SHARE
Beth Kindler
323 Hamilton Street
West Lafayette 47906
(317) 463-6605

IOWA

Bereavement Support Group
Richard Gilbert
Burlington Medical Center
618 N. Fourth Street, Room 1
Burlington 52601
(319) 753-3011

Grief Relief
Burlington Medical Center
Pastoral Care
602 N. Third
Burlington 52601
(319) 753-3395

*Parents With Empty Arms Support
    Group*
St. Luke's Hospital
Pastoral Care Department
1026 "A" Avenue, N.E.
Cedar Rapids 52402
(319) 369-7347

SHARE
Vicki and Steve Rall
807 W. Mills
Creston 50801
(515) 782-7752

Quad City SHARE
Anita Purcell
2128 Madison Street
Davenport 52804
(319) 322-2651

SHARE
G. Ferguson
Fort Madison Community Hospital
2210 Avenue H
Fort Madison 52627
(319) 372-6530

SHARE
Pat Williams
Mercy Hospital
500 Market Street
Iowa City 52245
(319) 339-3576

SHARE
Evan and Ann Terhorst
RR 2, Box 72
Ireton 51027
(712) 722-2079

Parent SHARE
Marjorie Evans
1001 E. Pennsylvania Avenue
Ottumwa 52501

SHARE
Cindy Myers/Tammi Guthmiller
1120 10th Street/1620 Oak Street
Sheldon 51201
(712) 324-4720/324-4272

Parents With Empty Arms
Sister Lou Marie Fidder, Chaplain,
    or Cathi Sesma, RN
Covenant Medical Center
3421 W. 9th
Waterloo 50702
(319) 236-4125

Parents Support Group
R. Striffler
St. Luke's Methodist Hospital
112 Jefferson Street
West Union 52175
(319) 422-3775

KANSAS

Bereaved Parents of Pittsburg
Howard Thompson
Quincy and Bypass
Pittsburg 66762

SHARE
Reverend Harry Tysen
c/o Asbury Hospital
400 South Santa Fe
Salina 67401
(913) 827-4411

*SHARE/Infant Loss Support Services,
    Inc.*
David and Janeice Rawles
P.O. Box 9516
Shawnee Mission 66201
(316) 322-2944, (913) 362-0902

KENTUCKY

Consoling Parents
Humana Hospital University
530 S. Jackson Street
Louisville 40202
(502) 589-4313

Consoling Parents
Francis E. Englander
1114 Hilliard Avenue
Louisville 40204
(502) 452-9138

Consoling Parents
c/o Dr. R. Wayne Willis
Alliant Health System
P.O. Box 35070
Louisville 40232-5070
(502) 629-6150

Norton Children's Hospital
Chaplain Wayne Willis
P.O. Box 35070
Louisville 40232

SHARE
Dorothy Van Sant
St. Anthony Hospital
Louisville 40204

Caring Friends
Judy Neal
Madisonville Medical Center
Hospital Drive
Madisonville 42431
(502) 825-5100

Compassionate Parents
Alice Higgins, Director of Patient
  Services
206 W. South Street
Mayfield 42066
(502) 247-5211

SHARE
P. Tuttle
Owensboro Daviess Hospital
P.O. Box 2799
Owensboro 42301
(502) 926-3030, Extension 117

Bereaved Parents Support Group
Anne Freeland
Western Baptist Hospital
Kentucky Avenue
Paducah 42001
(502) 898-8059, 575-2100

LOUISIANA

Infant Loss Support Group
Beth Manning, BCSW, ACSW
Women's Hospital
P.O. Box 95009
Baton Rouge 70895-9009
(504) 927-1300

SHARE
Humana Hospital
4200 Nelson Road
Lake Charles 70605
(318) 474-6370

Perinatal Bereavement Support Group
Ann Richardson, RNC
Ochsner Hospital
1516 Jefferson Highway
New Orleans 70121
(504) 838-3634

Resolve Through Sharing
Wendy Guichard, BCSW, ACSW,
  Social Services
Pendleton Methodist Hospital
5620 Read Boulevard
New Orleans 70127
(504) 244-5432

Shreveport-Bossier Chapter of SHARE
P. Thompson
Northwest State University
1800 Line Avenue
Shreveport 71101
(318) 677-3030, 929-2892

MAINE

Empty Arms (A SHARE Group)
Kathy Hobson
P.O. Box 104
Alna 04535
(207) 443-9425

MARYLAND

The Compassionate Friends
Anna Ruhrbaugh
44 River Drive
Annapolis 21403

The Compassionate Friends Infant Group
Debbie O'Connell
Harford County Group
1315 Mayflower Drive
Bel Air 21014
(301) 836-2252, 838-7417

Howard County SHARE
Maureen Dell
11868 Bright Passage
Columbia 21044

Sudden Infant Death Syndrome Alliance
Thomas L. Moran, President
10500 Little Patuxent Parkway, Suite 420
Columbia 21044
(800) 221-SIDS or (301) 964-8000

Labor of Love
Wendy Hite
Route 1, Box 139
Fairplay 21733
(301) 582-3697

National SIDS Foundation
Two Metro Plaza, Suite 205
8240 Professional Place
Landover 20785

MIS: Serving Metropolitan Washington, D.C., Maryland, and Virginia
Sharon Covington, LCSW
9715 Medical Center Drive #503
Rockville 20850
(301) 460-6222

MASSACHUSETTS

Clearinghouse of Mutual Help Groups Directory, 1991 Edition
c/o University of Massachusetts
112 Skinner Hall
Amherst 01003

Community Birth Loss Support Group
Patricia Cane
Auburn 01501
(508) 832-6985

Resolve, Inc.
P.O. Box 474
Belmont 02178

Center for Family Development
Intake Person
30 Tozer Road
Beverly 01915
(508) 922-3000, Extension 2630

Loss Support Group
Louise Hung, MSW, Social Service Department
Beverly Hospital
Herrick and Merrick Streets
Beverly 01915
(508) 922-3000, Extension 2710

Association of SIDS Program Professionals
c/o Massachusetts Center for SIDS
Mary McClain, RN, MS, President
Boston City Hospital
818 Harrison Avenue
Boston 02118
(617) 534-SIDS, 534-7437

COPE
530 Tremont Street
Boston 02116
(617) 357-5588

Family Support Center
295 Longwood Avenue
Boston 02115
(617) 232-8390

Massachusetts Chapter of SIDS Foundation
c/o Boston City Hospital
Penny Begley or Mary McClain, RNMS
818 Harrison Avenue
Boston 02118
(617) 534-7437 (24 hours)

Newborn Bereavement Support Group
Bernadette Reilly-Smorawski/Anne Armstrong
Ellison 3 NICU — Mass. General
Fruit Street
Boston 02114
(617) 726-3315

Parents' Group
c/o Brigham and Women's Hospital
Tamara May, MSW
75 Francis Street
Boston 02115
(617) 732-6462

SHARE
Jeanie Sullivan
87 Keddy Boulevard
Chicopee 01020
(413) 534-1526

*Compassionate Friends/Bereaved Parents
  of Central Middlesex County*
Concord
(508) 369-5105, (508) 897-9449

Neonatal Death Support Group
c/o Emerson Hospital
Paul Montgomery, Ph.D., and Sandi
  Grunwald, MSW
Old Road at Nine Acre Corner
Concord 01742
(508) 369-1400, Extension 1605

*C/SEC (Cesareans/Support, Education
  and Concern)*
15 Maynard Road
Dedham 02026

Bereaved Parents' Support Group
c/o St. Margaret's Hospital
Janet Leonard
90 Cushing Avenue
Dorchester 02125
(617) 436-8600, Extension 331

HOPE
Michelle Austin
23 Wampum Road
E. Falmouth 02536
(617) 337-7011, Extension 332

HOPE
Elaine Babineau
48 Place Road
Falmouth 02540
(508) 548-9603

HOPE
Nancy Twichell
Falmouth
(508) 540-3550

Pieta
2 Oak Street
Foxboro 02035
(508) 543-7956

Parent Bereavement Group
c/o Framingham Union Hospital
Mindy Shuster, MSW
Lincoln Street
Framingham 01701
(508) 879-7111, Extension 2356

*Bereavement Support Group of Franklin
  County*
Betty Thompson or Naomi Kendrick
Box 121
Greenfield 01302
(413) 773-7339 or 774-4637

SHARE
c/o Franklin Medical Center
Cynthia W. Kuusisto, LICSW
164 High Street
Greenfield 01301
(413) 772-0211, Extension 2303

Community Birth Loss Support Group
Fred and Wendy Wooden
Groton 01450
(508) 448-2567

SHARE
Jean Baxter
Hadley 01035
(413) 584-7097

Bereaved Parents' Group
Brian Dacey, LICSW
69 Summer Street
Haverhill 01830
(508) 372-8516

Pieta
Father William Wolkovich
14 Richard Road
Hudson 01749
(617) 762-0979

SHARE
c/o Cape Cod Hospital
Pat Mello or Kathy Alexander, RN
Hyannis 02601
(508) 771-1800, Extension 2156, or
  (508) 394-7827 (Tara)

HOPE
Kathy Kineen
Lawrence General Hospital
1 General Street
Lawrence 01842
(617) 683-4000, Extension 2550

*Safe Place (The Samaritans of Greater
    Lawrence)*
Margaret Serley
55 Jackson Street
Lawrence 01840
(508) 372-7200 (24 hours)

SHARE
Debby Wollwerth
Lenox
(413) 637-1633

The Compassionate Friends, Inc.
Sandi Sisitsky
48 Cobblestone Road
Longmeadow 01106
(413) 567-8705

*Perinatal Program, Greater Lynn
    Community M.H.C.*
Union Hospital
500 Lynnfield Street
Lynn 01940
(617) 598-8800, Extension 501
    (Barbara Wolf)

Birth Loss Support Group
Cheryl Oliveri
Milford 01757
(508) 473-1190, Extension 470

The Bereaved Parent Support Group
Cindy Gallup
Anna Jaques Hospital
25 Highland Avenue
Newburyport 01950
(508) 462-6600, Extension 294

BACE (Boston Assn. Childbirth Ed.)
Carole Kavanagh
Box 29
Newton 02160
(617) 244-5102

Childbirth Loss Group
c/o Newton-Wellesley Hospital
Department of Social Work and
    Continuing Care
2014 Washington Street
Newton 02162
(617) 243-6085

*The Compassionate Friends, North
    Shore/Boston Chapter*
Tom and Jean O'Hare
34 Lindor Road
North Reading 01864
(508) 644-4931

HOPE
c/o Norwood Hospital
Patricia Lang, RN
800 Washington Street
Norwood 02062
(617) 769-4000

Pieta
36 St. George Avenue
Norwood 02062
(508) 562-3016

Pieta
Mrs. Charlotte Baker
80 Hazelwood Drive
Norwood 02062
(617) 769-4185

REACH
c/o Berkshire Medical Center
Betty Jean Hydon, MSW
725 North Street, Social Services
    Department
Pittsfield 02101
(413) 499-4161, Extension 2422

HOPE
Valerie Corwin
Quincy 02164
(617) 659-2027

Resolve, Inc.
Massachusetts Chapter
P.O. Box 221
Sheldonville 02070
(617) 332-2579

Community Birth Loss Support Group
Carol Geary
P.O. Box 582
Shrewsbury 01545

Affinity
c/o Omega
Evelyn Gladu or Deborah Casey
270 Washington Street
Somerville 02143
(617) 625-1920 or 776-6396

SHARE
Jo-Ellen Height
South Lee
(413) 243-3413

HOPE
c/o South Shore Hospital
Sue Harrington, RN, BSN
55 Fogg Road
South Weymouth 02190
(617) 340-8368 or 340-8369

Bereavement Support Groups
Sister Mary Low Gillion or Office of
    Pastoral Ministry
625 Carew Street
Springfield 01104
(413) 732-3175, Extension 239

SHARE
Dashevsky
41 Churchill Street
Springfield 01108
(413) 736-3546

SHARE
Wanda Roberge
340 Dickinson Street
Springfield 01108

Resolve Through Sharing
c/o New England Memorial Hospital
Kelly Collier, RN, or Nancy Powell
5 Woodland Road
Stoneham 02180
(508) 657-8094 or (508) 369-0990

Loss
c/o Waltham West Medical Center
Paulette Melanson, RN
20 Hope Avenue
Waltham 02254
(617) 647-6308

Community Birth Loss Support Group
Merilyn Bambauer
West Boylston 01583
(508) 835-2130

Community Birth Loss Support Group
Kathy Marandqa
Whitinsville 01588
(508) 234-4363

HOPE
Pam or Rindy
Wilmington Health Center
Wilmington
(617) 273-2624 (Rindy) or (603)
    432-0069 (Pam)

HOPE
Barbara Bryant
Winchester Hospital
41 Highland Avenue
Winchester 01890
(617) 729-9000, Extension 3103 or
    3104

Community Birth Loss Support Group
c/o The Medical Center–Memorial
Elena Ann Coffey, LCSW
119 Belmont Street, Social Work
    Department
Worcester 01605
(508) 793-6286

Community Birth Loss Support Group
St. Vincent's Hospital
Claudia Neithercut, MSW, LICSW
25 Winthrop Street
Worcester 01604
(508) 798-6101

MICHIGAN

CARE
George and Kay Brown
304 S. Lane Street
Blissfield 49228
(517) 486-4102

*Pregnancy and Newborn Loss Support
    Group*
Ann Foley
Oakwood Hospital
18101 Oakwood Boulevard
Dearborn 48123-2500
(313) 593-7200

Resolve Through Sharing
Oakwood Hospital
Elaine Stoddard, RN Coordinator
18101 Oakwood Boulevard
Dearborn 48123-2500
(313) 593-7694

New Beginnings
Tom Zerbel
321 S. 15th Street
Escanaba 49819
(906) 786-2609

PEND
Butterworth Hospital NICU
Kim Wright, RN
100 Michigan Street, N.E.
Grand Rapids 49503
(616) 774-1523

Greater Holland Parent Grief Support Group
Karen North
Holland Community Hospital
602 Michigan Avenue
Holland 49423
(616) 392-5141

SHARE
Ruth Kavalherna, Neonatal
    Department
Bronson Hospital
Kalamazoo 49000
(616) 327-7844

HOPING
c/o Sparrow Hospital
Carolyn Wickham
P.O. Box 30480
Lansing 48909-9986
(517) 483-3873

HOPING
Mary Reed
1009 Robert Avenue
Mt. Pleasant 48858
(517) 773-6219

Friends Supporting Parents
Cindy Melitz
P.O. Box 206
Roseville 48066-0206
(313) 772-7293

"Looking Ahead . . ." Support Group
Deanna Duncan-Sarvis, MSW
Beaumont Hospital
3601 W. Thirteen Mile Road
Royal Oaks 48073
(313) 551-3160

HOPE
Judy O'Toole
Saginaw General Hospital
1447 N. Harrison
Saginaw 48602
(517) 771-4153, 771-4496

Bereaved Parents' Group
Marcia Boehm, ACSW, Social Work
    and Continuing Care Department
Providence Hospital
16001 W. Nine Mile Road, Box 2043
Southfield 48037
(313) 424-3113

Bereaved Parents
St. Bede's Church
Betty Rabaut
18290 W. Twelve Mile Road
Southfield 48076

Bereaved Parents' Support Group
Jeff and Sharon Wickey
63322 N. M.-66
Sturgis 49091

MINNESOTA

Mercy Hospital Grief Support Group
Gail Noller, LSW
4050 Coon Rapids Boulevard
Coon Rapids 55433-2586
(612) 422-4595

Parents' Grief Support Group
Barbara Elliott
4340 London Road
Duluth 55804
(218) 525-7268

St. Mary's Grief Support Center
Ben Wolfe, Director
407 E. Third Street
Duluth 55805
(218) 726-4402

SHARE
Denise Baker
906 S. Whitford
Fergus Falls 56537
(218) 736-2062

Friends Who Care
Jean Ruff
1011 Third Avenue, N.E.
Grand Rapids 55744
(218) 326-8876

Empty Arms
Ann and Dennis McCoy
772 Humphrey, Box 116
Lake Crystal 56055
(507) 726-6072

Empty Arms
Camille Koonce
126 W. 8th
Mankato 56001
(507) 387-2954

Grief Support Group
St. Mary's Hospital Hospice
C. Ceronsky
2414 S. 7th Street
Minneapolis 55454
(612) 337-4000

National Perinatal Bereavement Alliance
318 Groveland Avenue
Minneapolis 55403
(612) 870-1242

Perinatal Bereavement Support Group
Abbott/Northwestern Hospital
800 E. 28th Street
Minneapolis 55407
(612) 874-4428

Pregnancy After a Loss
Shari Perlman, MSW, LISW
4300 Manor Court Road
Minnetonka 55345
(218) 933-0713

Perinatal Death Support Group
Rochester Methodist Hospital
Kathryn Niesen, RN, MSN
201 West Center Street
Rochester 55901
(507) 286-7371

Empty Arms Infant Support Group
Alice Rademacher
349 38th Avenue North
St. Cloud 56303
(612) 253-1143

Children's Hospital
Jean London
Social Work Department
345 North Smith Avenue
St. Paul 55102
(612) 452-4110, 298-8720

Pregnancy and Infant Loss Center of Minnesota
Sherokee Ilse, Director
1415 W. Wayzata Boulevard #22
Wayzata 56560
(612) 473-9372, 292-1184 (24-hour Helpline)

Resolve Through Sharing
Marybeth Polus
P.O. Box 5600
Winona 55987
(507) 457-4345

MISSISSIPPI

Social Services Department
Boliver County Hospital
Highway 8E
Cleveland 38732

The Compassionate Friends
P.O. Box 20018
Jackson 39209
(601) 982-3363

MISSOURI

SHARE
Southeast Missouri Hospital
Linda Logan, RNC
1701 Lacey Street
Cape Girardeau 63701
(314) 651-5560

AMEND
Dianne Donahue
16043 Clarkson Woods Drive
Chesterfield 63017
(314) 532-3888

SHARE
Golden Valley Memorial Hospital
L. Jones
Junction Highway 7 and 13th North
Clinton 64735
(816) 885-5511, Extension 187, or
    696-2591

AMEND
Mrs. Peggy Springer
P.O. Box 174
Columbia 65201

EPS
Nancy Watrous
2410 N. Garth Avenue
Columbia 65201

The Compassionate Friends Infant Group
Judy Hanley
3065 Harness
Florissant 63033
(314) 837-4610

HOPE
P.O. Box 153
Florissant 63032

SHARE Infant Loss Support Services
Daren Archer
7402 E. 132nd Terrace
Grandview 64030
(816) 761-8890, 761-2333

Mothers in Crisis
c/o Freeman Hospital
Cheryl Rabe
1102 W. 32nd Street
Joplin 64804
(417) 623-2801

NAPSAC International
Route 1, Box 646
Marble Hill 63764
(314) 238-2010

AMEND
Maureen Connelly
4324 Berrywick Terrace
St. Louis 63128
(314) 487-7582

AMEND
Mary Wyss
9161 Rusticwood Trail
St. Louis 63126
(314) 843-3681

SHARE
St. Mary's Health Center
Karen Sutton
6420 Clayton Road
St. Louis 63117
(314) 768-8780

*The Compassionate Friends — Greater
    Ozark*
Pat Haas
4308 East Catalpa
Springfield 65809
(417) 882-6313

SHARE
Nancy Trombley
Box 222
Trenton 64683
(816) 359-3656

MONTANA

SHARE
Peggy Hanson
Janette Corp.
Northern Montana Hospital
Havre 59501
(406) 265-5200

NEBRASKA

*Alliance Pregnancy and Infant Loss
    Support Group*
Dee Przymus
HC 33, Box 14B
Alliance 69301
(308) 762-7419

The Compassionate Friends
T. Wielgus
Columbus Community Hospital
3111 19th Street
Columbus 68601
(402) 563-9632

Wee Care/Good Samaritan Hospital
Philip Gesseling, MD
Neonatal Intensive Care Unit
Kearney 68847
(308) 236-4541

Bridges
c/o St. Elizabeth Hospital
Joanne Bronson or Karen Liechti
555 South 70th
Lincoln 68510
(402) 486-7070

HOPE
Centering Corporation
Dr. S. Marv and Joy Johnson
4902 Happy Hollow Boulevard,
   Box 3367
Omaha 68103-0367
(402) 553-1200

HOPE
First Christ Church
6630 Dodge Street
Omaha 68132
(402) 558-1939

*Pregnancy and Infant Loss Support
   Group*
Barb Hill
HC 65, Box 25
Wauneta 69045
(308) 882-4002

NEW HAMPSHIRE

*Pregnancy Loss and Early Infant Death
   Support Group*
Sharon Walker, MS
380 Roxbury Road
Marlborough 03455
(603) 876-4495

*HOPE of Wilmington Regional Health
   Center*
Pam Bureau
35 Blossom Road
Windham 03087
(603) 432-0069

NEW JERSEY

*Englewood Hospital Pregnancy Loss
   Support Group*
Sue Dziemian
350 Engle Street, Englewood 07631,
   or 22 Turnure Street, Bergenfield
   07621
(201) 384-8258

*HOPING of Hackettstown Community
   Hospital*
Beth Van Meter
651 Willoco Grove Street
Hackettstown 07840
(908) 852-5100

St. Barnabas Perinatal Bereavement
Dorothy Kurzweil, MSW
Old Short Hills Road
Livingston 07039
(201) 533-5745

SHARE
Monmouth Medical Center
Kay Peterson
300 Second Avenue
Long Branch 07740
(201) 222-5200, Extension 3399

PRIDE
Jersey Shore Medical Center
Kate Luscombe Elliott, RNC
1945 Route 33
Neptune 07754
(908) 776-4316

MIDS
Marsha Silbert Dreier
373 Crosson Place
North Plainfield 07063
(201) 668-0085

MIDS, Inc. — Support Group
Janet Tischler
16 Crescent Drive
Parsippany 07054
(201) 263-6730

HOPE
Our Lady of Fatima Church
E. Forte
499 New Market Road
Piscataway 08854
(201) 968-5555

UNITE, Inc.
Mary Wallace/Eileen Stewart, RN
Medical Center
Princeton 08540
(609) 896-2941 (Eileen), or (201)
    359-7812 (Mary)

Friends of Parents
Salem County Memorial Hospital
Salem 08079
(609) 935-4357

HOPE
Marsha and Ed Roger
314 Salem Court
Somerville 08876
(201) 722-7726

Miscarriage Support Group
Bonnie Phillips
Methodist Church
Bethel Road
Somers Point 08244
(609) 927-9294

SHARE
Marge Dempseyl
43 E. Shore Trail
Stockholm 07460
(201) 697-2178

MIDS — Bergen County Chapter
Pam Tyler
Holy Name Hospital School of
    Nursing
Teaneck 07666
(201) 864-3867

Empty Arms
John F. Kennedy Memorial Hospital
Hurffville–Cross Keys Road
Turnersville 08012
(609) 589-3300

HELP
Eileen Thompson
607 North Oxford Avenue
Ventnor 08706
(609) 822-5265

The Compassionate Friends
Pat Turoczy
P.O. Box 63
Verona 07044
(201) 857-2464

Helping Hands
c/o Newcomb Hospital
Judith Schmeelk-Ford
65 South State Street
Vineland 08360
(609) 691-9000, Extension 6179

HOPING of West Jersey Hospital
Janet Millspaugh, RN, BS, CCE,
    Director of Community Health
    Education
101 Carnie Boulevard
Voorhees 08043
(609) 772-5576

MIDS Support Group of Passaic County
Cindy DeRosa
51 Vreeland Road
West Milford 07480
(201) 728-2998

Bereavement Group
Pascack Valley Hospital
Lori Postal
Old Hook Road
Westwood 07675-3181
(201) 690-0441

HOPING of South Jersey
Zurbrugg Memorial Hospital
Susan Skelly
Rancocas Valley Division
Willingboro 08046

NEW MEXICO

SHARE
Trinity Lutheran Church
Ida Turner, Secretary
Box 1113
Hobbs 88240
(505) 392-5407

NEW YORK

EASE
Albany Medical Center
Linda Raydo
New Scotland Avenue, Room E501
Albany 12208
(518) 383-2943

SHARE
St. Peter's Hospital
Reverend Paula J. Gravelle
315 S. Manning Boulevard
Albany 12208
(518) 454-1602

Sharing Parents
St. Mary's, Wellness Institute
Sister Rita Jean DuBrey, RN, MSN
427 Guy Park Avenue
Amsterdam 12010
(518) 842-1900

SHARE of Genesee County
Genesee Memorial Hospital
Joan LaFever, RN
127 North Street
Batavia 14020
(716) 344-5242

Bereavement Support Group
Lourdes Hospital
Kathi DiFulvio, CSW
169 Riverside Drive
Binghamton 13905
(607) 798-5692

Bereavement Clinics
Kings County Hospital
Nancy O'Donahue
451 Clarkson Avenue
Brooklyn 11203
(201) 857-2464

Grief Groups
Dr. Roberta Temes
262 Coleridge Street
Brooklyn 11235
(718) 646-5537

Neonatal Bereavement
SUNY/Health Science Center
Sharon S. Pantel, CSW, or Eva
 Beller, MS
450 Clarkson Avenue
Brooklyn 11203-2908
(718) 270-1189 or 270-2072

Perinatal Bereavement Group
Mercy Hospital
Pastoral Care Department
1000 N. Village Avenue
Brooklyn 11571
(718) 255-2241

SHARE
Kathleen M. Huffer
6080 Rose Arbor Lane
Cicero 13039
(315) 458-8081

St. Mary's Bereavement Ministry
Mrs. Carol Carney
East Islip
(516) 277-4759

Lost Miracles
St. Adalbert Parish
Arlene Campisi or G. Debiase
52-20 84th Street
Elmhurst 11373
(718) 639-0212

SHARE
Lois Sugarman
6726 Gleason Place
Fayetteville 13066
(315) 446-1262

EASE
Kris Clements
P.O. Box 2223
Glens Falls 12801
(518) 587-7904

SHARE
Queens Hospital Center
R. Hoffman, RN, or T. Locilent, RN
82-68 164 Street
Jamaica 11432
(718) 990-2551 or 990-2838

Crisis Support Group
UHS Wilson Hospital
Lorraine Lee, RN
3357 Harris Street
Johnson City 13790
(607) 770-6101

Help with Emotions After Pregnancy Loss
Kathy Meritheu
113 N. Woodland Drive
Liverpool 13088
(315) 457-9623

Bereavement and Loss Center of New York
Anne Rosberger, MSW, CSW, or
   Henry Rosberger, MD
170 E. 83 Street, Suite 4P
New York 10028
(212) 879-5655

National Council of Jewish Women of New York
Ingrid Kohn, CSW, Coordinator
537 West 121st Street, Apartment 56
New York 10027

Pregnancy Loss Support Program
Amy Gershenson
9 East 69th Street
New York 10021
(212) 535-5900, Extension 10

St. Philip's Bereavement Ministry
Cindy Pinto
Northport
(516) 261-0495

Together Loss of a Child
Laurie Britt
29 S. White Street
Poughkeepsie 12601
(914) 473-7795

Mercy Hospital
Pastoral Care Department
1000 N. Village Avenue
Rockville Centre 11570
(516) 255-2241

Infant Bereavement Group
Mary Wasacz, MS, RN, CS
172 Madison Road
Scarsdale 10583
(914) 725-1060

SHARE
Staten Island Hospital
Sandra Dolan, RN, Nursery
475 Seaview Avenue
Staten Island 10305
(718) 390-9797

NORTH CAROLINA

SHARE
Stanley Memorial Hospital
OB Department
Albermarle 28001
(704) 463-7894

Kinder-Mourn, Inc.
6900 Percade Lane
Charlotte 28215

Bereaved Parents
Triangle Hospice
Margaret S. Miles, RN, Ph.D.
3605 Shannon Road
Durham 27707
(919) 942-8597

Families with Healing Hearts
Robin L. Kivett, RNC, NP
4042 Pleasant View Drive
Fayetteville 28301
(919) 485-7181

SHARE of Wayne County
Lu Saulmon
P.O. Box 10303
Goldsboro 27530
(919) 735-7043

AMEND
Susan Ridenour
1711 Independence Road
Greensboro 24708

Comfort
The Women's Hospital of
   Greensboro
Terri Burleson, RN, Nurse Manager
801 Green Valley Road
Greensboro 27408
(919) 691-6900

SHARE
Pitt County Memorial Hospital
Donna Weeks or Linda Roy
P.O. Box 6028
Greenville 27834

PROP
Senior Chaplain
Naval Hospital
Jacksonville 28542
(919) 451-4070

SHARE of Avery County
Janet E. Johnson
P.O. Box 970
Newland 28657
(704) 733-3539

TLC
Jeri Conner
Route 4, Box 161-A
Rutherfordton 28139
(704) 248-2261

NORTH DAKOTA

Aid in Infant Death
Mary Jo Horsager
Lutheran Social Services
1325 11th Street, South
Fargo 58102
(701) 235-7341

The Compassionate Friends of FM Area
Syl and Marge Loegering
Box 389
Fargo 58107
(701) 235-7341, 282-8714

SHARE
Community Memorial Hospital
Joey Belling, MS, RD
Route 2, Box 124
Hettinger 58639
(701) 567-4561

SHARE Support Team
Darlene Frey or Diane Heupel
RR1, Box 79, Mott 58646, or RR1,
    Box 89, New Leipzig 58562
(701) 584-2661

OHIO

Bereaved Parents' Support Group
3136 Ellet Avenue
Akron 44312

Solace
St. Paul's Catholic Church
433 Mission Drive
Akron 44301

SHARE
Ruth Detchon
Route 1
Amsterdam 43903
(614) 543-3264

HOPE
Georgia Kohart
400 Vine Street
Archbold 73502
(419) 445-1602

Parents Helping Parents — SHARE
Connie Harmon
33803 Electric E2
Avon Lake 44012
(216) 933-7150

SHARE
Linda Stratton
3550 SR 47 West
Bellefontaine 43311

SHARE
Marilyn Miller Graef
1272 Indian Hill Drive
Bolivar 44612
(216) 874-3100

Cincinnati HOPING
Karen Young
1007 Windzag
Cincinnati 45242

For Fathers of Children Who've Died
Reverend Ken Czillinger
St. Matthias'
1044 West Kempner Road
Cincinnati 45240
(513) 851-1930

Greater Cincinnati/Northern Kentucky
    SIDS Chapter
Beverly Stewart
College of Medicine
231 Bethesda Avenue, Room 6153
Cincinnati 45267-0541
(513) 559-8000

Mothers of Children Who've Died
Ruth Donnelly
685 Lullaby Court
Cincinnati 45238
(513) 451-3022

Mothers of Children Who've Died
Connie Baron
793 Carini Lane
Cincinnati 45218
(513) 825-3089

Mothers Supporting Mothers
Pat Stetter
5890 Fourson Drive
Cincinnati 45238
(513) 922-7896

Parents' Support Groups
Father Ken Czillinger
IHM Church
7820 Beechmont Avenue
Cincinnati 45230
(513) 474-5570

PAT/Family Counsel
Sister Joan Carole Schaffner, ACSW
Good Samaritan Hospital
3217 Clifton Avenue
Cincinnati 45220-2489
(513) 872-1400

Reach Out to Grieving Parents
Carole Bonno
902 Seton Avenue
Cincinnati 45205
(513) 921-7690

FEEL
c/o Fairview General Hospital
Linda DiPasquale
18101 Lorain Avenue
Cleveland 44111-5856
(216) 476-7000

PEND
Rainbow Babies' and Children's
  Hospital
2101 Adelbert Road
Cleveland 44106
(216) 844-3754

*Parents' Group Coping with Perinatal
  Loss/SIDS*
Nancy Thomas, RN
Children's Medical Center
1 Children's Plaza
Dayton 45404-1815
(513) 226-8300

SHARE
Miami Valley Hospital, Perinatal
  Health Center
Brenda Nickells, RNC, BSN
1 Wyoming Street
Dayton 45409
(513) 223-6192, Extension 3650

Parents Who Share
Jim and Jane Linbon
1573 Westgate Drive
Defiance 43512

Share the Loss
Marilyn M. Melison, RNC
Euclid General Hospital
101 East 185th Street
Euclid 44119
(216) 531-9000, Extension 227

Parent Support
Childbirth Education Association
Linda Baily
2183 Larchdale
Guy Falls 44221

CARE
June Henderson
4300 Leffler Drive
Lima 45806
(419) 999-3415

Remember Me
Janet Osborne, RN, CNT
St. Charles Hospital
2600 Navarre Avenue, Oregon
  43616, or 702 Weston Street,
  Toledo 43609
(419) 698-7462 or 385-6524

SHARE/Lake County/Lake East Hospital
Obstetrics Department or Social
  Services
Washington at Liberty Street
Painesville 44077
(216) 354-2400

Feelings After . . .
Attn: Family Life
Donna Naso, RN
7007 Powers Boulevard
Parma 44129
(216) 888-1800, Extension 4031

SHARE
Cheryl Holton
8132 Weaver Road, N.E.
St. Louisville 43071

CARE
Dr. Irwin Weinfeld, MD
Center for Women and Children
2142 North Cove Boulevard
Toledo 43606
(419) 473-4218 (Hospital Operator)

Friends Supporting Parents
C. Shelhart, RN, or K. Brzuchalski,
  RN
Riverside Hospital
1600 North Superior Street
Toledo 43604
(419) 729-6000, Extension 6416

Parents Reach Out
Betty Teall, RN
St. Vincent's Medical Center
2213 Cherry Street
Toledo 43608
(419) 321-2856

SHARE
c/o Trumbull Memorial Hospital
Patricia Lauer, RN, BSN,
  Educational Services Department
1350 East Market Street
Warren 44482-1269
(216) 841-9880

HOPE
c/o Fulton County Health Center
Connie Kloppenhofer, RN
725 South Shoop Avenue
Wauseon 43567
(419) 335-2015, Extension 2350

SHARE
Susan P. Sulzer, RN
St. John West Shore Hospital
29000 Center Ridge Road
West Lake 44145
(216) 835-6094

HEAL
Sister Jean Orsuto, RN, MSN
St. Elizabeth Hospital Medical Center
1044 Belmont Avenue
Youngstown 44501
(216) 746-7211, page, or Extension
  3105

OKLAHOMA

*The Compassionate Friends/Norman
  Chapter*
Betty Smith
4400 West Main, Box 120
Norman 73072
(405) 329-4280 or 360-4287

PRIDE
Joan E. Morehead, LPN
Norman Regional Hospital
901 N. Porter, Box 1308
Norman 73070
(405) 321-1700, Extension 3500 or
  1015

The Compassionate Friends
Cheryl Hille
7205 Crown Point Road
Oklahoma City 73132
(405) 670-1159

PRIDE
Connie Furrh, RN
5501 N. Portland
Oklahoma City 73112
(405) 949-6399

PRIDE
C. Boatright, L. Wulz, RN
Mercy Hospital
4300 West Memorial Road
Oklahoma City 73120
(405) 752-3763 or 752-3784

AMEND
Cindy Wilcox
1344 E. 26th Place
Tulsa 74100

OREGON

Perinatal Loss
Pat Schwiebert, RN
2116 N.E. 18
Portland 97212
(503) 284-7426

Parents Supporting Parents
Judy Klier
17345 S.W. Thistlebrook
Tigard 97224
(503) 620-0936

PENNSYLVANIA

SHARE
Thelma Garrett, MSW, Social
Services
Abington Memorial Hospital
1200 Old York Road
Abington 19001
(215) 576-2570

SHARE of Altoona Hospital
Jane Callan
620 Howard Avenue
Altoona 16601
(814) 949-3146

Parents' Support Group
c/o Social Services
Deborah Lewis Melone
Bryn Mawr Hospital
Bryn Mawr 19010
(215) 896-3214

HOPE
Oskana Leader, RN
Box 934
Chambersburg 17201-0934
(717) 264-5171 or 264-1025

SHARE (Washington PA Group)
Patti Mounts
Route 1, Box 260
Clayville 15232
(412) 948-3842

Empty Arms
Julia Howell
Geisinger Medical Center
N. Academy Avenue
Danville 17821
(717) 271-6567

UNITE (Fitzgerald Mercy Hospital)
Krista Russel, Social Services
Lansdowne Avenue and Baily Road
Darby 19023
(215) 237-4750

Mary Ann Egges
10 Highland Court
Downington 19335
(215) 269-9606

Empty Arms, Inc.
Patty McGuinness
6416 Wyndham Court
Erie 16505
(814) 838-6346

The Compassionate Friends/Parents of Infants
Mary Kay Steele
RD #1
Falls Creek 15840
(814) 375-1045

Capital Area SHARE
Suzanne Woods
P.O. Box 2521
Harrisburg 17105
(717) 236-5999

SHARE
Barbara Antinora
Lee Hospital
320 Main Street
Johnstown 15901
(814) 533-0201

SHARE/Northeast Pennsylvania
Judith M. Nowak, RN, Technical
Adviser
Nesbitt Memorial Hospital
562 Wyoming Avenue, Department
of Community Relations
Kingston 18704
(717) 288-1411, Extension 4024

SHARE of Lancaster
Sheryl Cushman
P.O. Box 961
Lancaster 17604
(717) 396-9613

SHARE
Nancy Sauder
P.O. Box 961
Lancaster 17603
(717) 396-9613

UNITE of Lower Bucks County
Katie Popp, RN
St. Mary's Hospital
Langhorne-Newton Road
Langhorne 19047
(215) 750-2118

SHARE
Beverly Clark, RN
Lebanon Valley General Hospital
4th and Willow Streets
Lebanon 17042
(717) 273-8521

SHARE of the Lehigh Valley
Faye Dorney-Magitz
221 Willow Street
Macungie 18062
(215) 966-3891

SHARE of the Lehigh Valley
Kathy Kuhn
RD #1, Box B54
New Tripoli 18066
(215) 285-6144

Empty Arms
Andrea Martz
P.O. Box 212
Oneida 18242
(717) 384-3790

Pennsylvania SIDS Center
Rosanne English, RN, PA
Thomas Jefferson University
834 Chestnut Street, Suite 200
Philadelphia 19107
(215) 222-1400 or (800) 258-SIDS

*UNITE, Inc., Grief Support after Death
    of a Baby*
Janis Heil, M.Ed., Director
c/o Social Services
7600 Central Avenue
Philadelphia 19111
(215) 728-3777

Pregnancy Loss Group
Medical Social Work Department
Magee Women's Hospital
300 Halket Street
Pittsburgh 15213
(201) 647-4255

SHARE
Carmen Anderson
5081 Rosecrest Drive
Pittsburgh 15201
(412) 362-8670

SHARE
Andrea F. Joubert
Allegheny General Hospital
320 E. North Avenue, Lifestages 6th
    Floor, South Tower
Pittsburgh 15236
(412) 655-1272

Resolve Through Sharing
Diane Carp
Grand View Hospital
700 Lawn Avenue
Sellersville 18960
(215) 453-4902

Pregnancy Loss Support Group
Nancy L. Grandovic, RN
Blackburn Road
Sewickley 15143-1498
(412) 749-7201

SHARE of Washington
Patricia M. Mounts
P.O. Box 1315
Washington 15301
(415) 948-3842

*Tioga County Bereaved Parents' Support
    Group*
Kaye Galloway
31 Meade Street
Wellsboro 16901
(717) 724-5329

SHARE
J. Nowak, RN, M. Gross
Mercy Hospital
360 Canal Street
Wilkes-Barre 18634
(717) 826-3100 or 826-3682

SHARE of York, Pennsylvania
Rose Marie Stein/Marilyn Gross
1305 Fairlane Drive
York 17404
(717) 845-4370

SOUTH CAROLINA

Perinatal Loss Support Team
Cheryl Hale, RN
Trident Medical Center
9330 Medical Plaza Drive
Charleston 29418
(803) 797-8805

CARING
Elaine Fant
Richland Memorial Hospital
5 Richland Medical Park
Columbia 29203
(803) 765-7601

SHARE of Newberry
Biff Riebe
66 Nance Street
Newberry 29108
(803) 276-3672

SOUTH DAKOTA

Bereaved Parents' Group
Mary Reshara
324 St. Anne Street
Rapid City 57701

Families/Stillborn Child
Doug Soule and Mary Weigelt
800 East 21st Street (School of
    Medicine)
University of South Dakota
Sioux Falls 57101
(605) 339-6785

SHARE
Sharon Stratman
Sacred Heart Hospital
501 Summit
Yankton 57078
(605) 665-9371

TENNESSEE

Grief Support Team
Cynthia Spears, RN, Obstetric
    Education
Erlanger Medical Center
975 East Third Street
Chattanooga 37403
(615) 778-6103

The Compassionate Friends Infant Group
Barbara Heflin, Social Work Services
Memorial Hospital
Clarksville 37043-3160
(615) 552-6622

*PEPD (Parents Experiencing Perinatal
    Death)*
Barbara Turner
P.O. Box 38445
Germantown 38138
(901) 372-5102

HOPING
Diane Hawking, RN
Holston Valley Hospital
Kingsport 37662

SHARE
Don Ferguson
Fort Saunders Med. Reg. Center
1901 Clinch Avenue, S.W.
Knoxville 37916
(615) 546-2811

SHARING
Derenda Hodge, RN, CNS
Vanderbilt University Hospital
D2120 MCN
Nashville 37232-2410
(615) 322-5000

TEXAS

Empty Cradle
Linda Watson
P.O. Box 171492
Arlington 76003
(817) 572-0875 or 478-5812
(L. Lambreth)

SHARE
Chaplain Eric Smith
Harris Methodist H.E.B. Hospital
1600 Hospital Parkway
Bedford 76022
(817) 685-4848

COPE's Angels
Tina Kurtz
1913 Thames
Corpus Christi 78413
(512) 992-2661, Extension 512, or
    992-3954 (Tina)

Marie Okerson
12622 Pine Bough
Cypress 77429
(713) 373-0105

Parent to Parent
Sharon Whitney, ACSW
Fort Worth Children's Hospital
1400 Cooper
Fort Worth 76104
(817) 336-9861

*HAND (Houston's Aid in Neonatal
    Death)*
Iris Fisherman
6413 Vanderbilt
Houston 77005
(713) 667-1250

SHARE
Sharon Cook, ACSW
1114 Wind Song
Longview 75604
(714) 297-0005

SHARE
Raymond Wolfe/Ann Allison
c/o Methodist Hospital
P.O. Box 1201
Lubbock 79408-9954
(806) 793-4027

SHARE
Constance Clear, CSW-ACP BCD
3534 Avenue B
San Antonio 78209
(512) 822-4135

HAND
Mrs. Karen Riley
3115 Stephens Creek Lane
Sugarland 77478
(713) 980-7496

UTAH

SHARE
Susan Ericksen
Logan Regional Hospital
1400 N. 500 East
Logan 84321
(801) 753-4377

SHARE
McKay Dee Hospital/St. Benedict's
    Hospital
Margaret Wardle
610 W. Elberta
Ogden 84404
(801) 782-5599

SHARE
Cynthia Gaufin
786 E. Redford Drive
Provo 84604
(801) 225-8001

SHARE
Heidi Stevens
Dixie Medical Center
1419 W. 490 N.
St. George 84770

SHARE — Parents of Utah
Christine Balderas
3118 S. 2850 E.
Salt Lake City 84109
(801) 486-9804 or 942-3199

Sharing Heart
Thomas D. Coleman
University of Utah Medical Center
50 N. Medical Drive, Pediatrics
    2B425
Salt Lake City 84132

VERMONT

Reach Out
Susan Alward
No. Co. Hospital
Prouty Drive, RFD #2
Newport 05855
(802) 334-7331, Extension 269

VIRGINIA

*Pregnancy Loss/Infant Death Resource
   Group*
Linda White
Route 4, Box Al, Hillman Highway
Abingdon 24210
(703) 628-7721 or 628-2533

MIS
Linda Juret
6486 Crayford Street
Burke 22015
(703) 455-2877

*The Compassionate Friends of Central
   Virginia*
Barbara Dimmick
121 Sailview Drive
Forest 24551
(804) 525-6473

SHARE
Carol Mason
Mary Washington Hospital
14 Ridgemore Circle
Fredericksburg 22405
(703) 371-3158

SHARE
Jeanie Flinn, Social Worker
John Randolph Hospital
700 N. Fourth, P.O. Box 971
Hopewell 23860
(804) 541-7494

Perinatal Loss Support Group
P.O. Box 1284
Manassas 22110

SHARE
Susan Finelli, Labor and Delivery
Mary Immaculate Hospital
800 Denbigh Boulevard
Newport News 23602
(804) 599-5453

SHARE
DePaul Hospital
Angela Gusky
150 Kingsley Lane
Norfolk 23505
(804) 889-5000

SHARE
Linda Bennington, RNC
Virginia Beach General Hospital
1060 First Colonial Road
Virginia Beach 23454
(804) 481-8292

WASHINGTON

Parents of Prematures
Lauri Lowen, President
13613 N.E. 26th Place
Bellevue 98005
(206) 883-6040

Parents of Stillborns
Everett General Hospital
1321 Colby Street
Everett 98201
(206) 259-3384 (Cynthia); 347-3437
   (Mary); 659-9615 (Nancy)

HOPING of Olympia
Susan and Don St. George
413 N. Lilly Road
Olympia 98506
(206) 459-4412

Parents of Stillborns
Judy Campbell
Group Health Coop, East Side
Redmond 98073

Birth and Life Bookstore
7001 Alonzo Avenue, N.W.
P.O. Box 70625
Seattle 98107-0625
(206) 789-4444

P.S.: A Parents' Support Group
Sharon Moody, President
P.O. Box 17451
Seattle 98107-1269
(206) 782-0054

P.S. My Baby Died
Carla D. Curtis, Secretary
3509 N.E. 33rd Street
Tacoma 98422
(206) 838-9833

Tacoma Parents of Stillborns
Tacoma General Hospital
315 S. K Street
Tacoma 98422
(206) 659-9615

Pregnancy Loss Support Group
Linda Stepniewski
Route #2, Box 2242
Wapato 98951
(509) 877-6424

Resolve Through Sharing
Kay Long, Jensea Haslett, or Kent
  Roberts
Yakima Memorial Hospital
2811 Tieton Drive
Yakima 98902
(509) 575-8000

WEST VIRGINIA

SHARE
Susan Spagnuolo
242 Gordon
Bridgeport 26330
(304) 842-6802

SHARE
Donna McCartney
Route 12, Box 298
Morgantown 26505
(304) 296-5667

WISCONSIN

The Compassionate Friends
Pat Vernier
Maple Lane Road
Ashland 54806
(715) 682-3818

Bereavement Persons Group
Carol Garner or Laurie Brown
St. Mary's Hospital
707 South Mills Street
Barron 54812
(715) 537-9056

HOPE
Vicki Jentoft-Johnson
Our Savior's Lutheran Church
749 Bluff Street
Beloit 53511
(608) 362-2623

Resolve Through Sharing
Anne Henning, SW
Beloit Memorial Hospital
1969 W. Hart Road
Beloit 53511
(608) 364-5130

SHARE
Patty Williams
Route #2, Highway 81, Box 124
Beloit 53511
(608) 365-1392

Resolve Through Sharing
Sandy Giacommona
Luther Hospital
1405 Babcock
Eau Claire 54701
(715) 839-3169, Extension 3169, or
  835-2858

SHARE
Sacred Heart Hospital
900 W. Clairemont Avenue
Eau Claire 54701
(715) 839-4121

Resolve Through Sharing
Patricia Weidman
St. Agnes Hospital
430 E. Division Street
Fond du Lac 54935
(414) 929-1800

The Compassionate Friends
Barbara Stellmacher
1081 Van Dyne Road
Fond du Lac 54935
(414) 922-5467

SHARE
Char Buelow, Social Services
  Department
St. Vincent's Hospital
P.O. Box 13508
Green Bay 54307
(414) 433-8261

Parents Caring
Phyllis Rozinski
St. Catherine's Hospital
3556 7th Avenue
Kenosha 53140-1490
(414) 656-3316

Resolve Through Sharing
Bonnie K. Gensch, RN
Lutheran Hospital
1910 South Avenue, 6th Floor
  Maternity
LaCrosse 54601
(608) 785-0530, Extension 3796

SHARE
Karen Olson, RN
St. Francis Medical Center
700 West Avenue South
La Crosse 54601
(608) 785-0940

Bereaved Parents' Support Group
Pat Krantz
3276 Maple Grove Drive
Madison 53719
(608) 845-9322

Bereavement
Sister M. Mulcady
St. Mary's Hospital
707 South Mills Street
Madison 53715
(608) 251-6100

TLC
Patient and Family Services
St. Joseph's Hospital
611 St. Joseph Avenue
Marshfield 54449
(715) 387-7890

Ray of Hope
Valerie Babcock
Tri-County M.H. Center
111 Mills Street
Mauston 53948
(608) 847-5488

Resolve Through Sharing
Chris Van Mullem
Mt. Sinai Medical Center
950 N. 12th
Milwaukee 53233
(414) 289-8200

Resolve Through Sharing
Maureen Smentek, Coordinator
St. Francis Hospital
3237 S. 16th Street
Milwaukee 53221
(414) 647-5000

Resolve Through Sharing
Cheryl Jaeger
St. Michael's Hospital
2400 W. Villard
Milwaukee 53209-4999
(414) 527-8000, Beep 228

The Compassionate Friends
Sherry Nutcher
114 Woodside Court
Neenah 54956
(414) 729-6375

Theda Clark Regional Medical Center
Marshelle Bergstrom, RN, MS
130 2nd Street
Neenah 54953
(414) 729-3100

The Compassionate Friends
Ann-Marie Luker
St. Peter's Church
345 High Avenue
Oshkosh 54901

Parents' Group
Marsha Fritsche, RN
Prairie du Chien Memorial Hospital
705 East Taylor Street
Prairie du Chien 53821
(608) 326-2431

Parents Sharing
LuAn Wells
St. Luke's Hospital
1320 Wisconsin Avenue
Racine 53403
(414) 636-2790

SHARE
St. Nicholas Hospital
1601 N. Taylor Drive
Sheboygan 53081
(414) 459-4624

Bereaved Parents' Group
Dick and Donna Clesigen
St. Michael's Hospital
911 Illinois Avenue
Stevens Point 54481

Parents Supporting Parents
Mary Berg, RN
Rice Clinic
2501 Main Street
Stevens Point 54481

Resolve Through Sharing
Lynn Carey, MSN, RN
Waukesha Memorial Hospital
725 American Avenue
Waukesha 53186
(414) 544-2252

SAID
Joel and Rae Ann Sigel
409 Lake View Drive
Wausau 54401
(715) 842-0237

Consoling Friends
Patti Luedtke, Medical Social Worker
551 Silverbrook Drive
West Bend 53095
(414) 334-5533

Organizations Outside the United States

CANADA

The Canadian Foundation for the Study of Infant Deaths
586 Eglinton Avenue East, Suite 308
Toronto, ON MP4 1P2
(416) 488-3260

The Compassionate Friends
National Center
685 William Avenue
Winnipeg, MB R3E OZ2
(204) 787-2460

THE UNITED KINGDOM

The Compassionate Friends
6 Denmark Street
Bristol BS1 5DQ
England
(0272) 292-778

The Foundation for the Study of Infant Deaths
35 Belgrave Square
London SW1X 8QB
England
(071) 235-0965
(071) 235-1721

Irish Sudden Infant Death Association
Carmichael House
4 North Brunswick Street
Dublin 7
Ireland
(010) 3531-747007

Miscarriage Association
c/o Clayton Hospital, Northgate
Wakefield WF1 3JS
West Yorks, England

SANDS (Stillbirth And Neonatal Death Society)
28 Portland Place
London W1N 4DE
England
(071) 436-5881

Scottish Cot Death Trust
Royal Hospital for Sick Children
Yorkhill, Glasgow G3 8SJ
Scotland
(041) 357-3946

Adoption Resources

National Adoption Hotline
(202) 328-8072

FAIR (Families Adopting Inter-Racially)
98 Woodland
Menlo Park
CA 94025

AASK (Aid to the Adoption of Special
 Kids)
3530 Grand Avenue
Oakland
CA 94611
(415) 451-1748

Adopt International
(for California residents only)
3142 La Mesa Drive
San Carlos
CA 94070
(415) 593-1008

International Concerns Committee for
 Children
911 Cypress Drive
Boulder
CO 80303
(303) 494-8333

FCVN (Friends of Children of Various
 Nations)
1818 Gaylord Street
Denver
CO 80206
(303) 321-8251

National Adoption Information
 Clearinghouse
1400 I Street, N.W.
Suite 600
Washington
D.C. 20005
(202) 842-1919

NCFA (National Committee For
 Adoption)
1930 17th Street, N.W.
Washington
D.C. 20009
(202) 328-1200

FACE (Families Adopt Children
 Everywhere)
Northwood Station
P.O. Box 28058
Baltimore
MD 21239

Project Impact
25 West Street
Boston
MA 02111
(617) 451-1472

SPACE (Single Parents Adopt Children
 Everywhere)
6 Sunshine Avenue
Natick
MA 01760
(508) 655-5426

Open Door Society
130 Temple Street
West Newton
MA 02165
(617) 527-5660

Adoptive Families of America, Inc.
3333 Highway 100 North, Suite 203
Minneapolis
MN 55422
(612) 535-4829

NACAC (North American Council on
 Adoptable Children)
P.O. Box 14808
Minneapolis
MN 55414
(612) 625-0330

National Adoption Center
1218 Chestnut Street
2nd Floor
Philadelphia
PA 19107
(215) 925-0200

Intercountry Adoption
WACAT
P.O. Box 88948
Seattle
WA 98138
(206) 575-4550

Bibliography

THE EMOTIONAL AND PHYSICAL IMPACT OF LOSING A PREGNANCY

Becker, Ernest. *The Denial of Death.* New York: The Free Press, 1975.

Benedek, Therese. "The Psychobiology of Pregnancy." In *Parenthood: Its Psychology and Psychopathology,* ed. James Anthony and Theresa Benedek. Boston: Little, Brown, 1970.

Bibring, Grete L. *Some Considerations of the Psychological Processes in Pregnancy. Psychoanalytic Study of the Child,* vol. 14. New York: International University Press, 1959.

Bibring, Grete L., T. F. Dwyer, D. S. Huntington, and A. F. Valenstein. "A Study of the Psychological Processes in Pregnancy and of the Earliest Mother-Child Relationship. I. Some Propositions and Comments." In *Psychoanalytic Study of the Child,* vol. 16. New York: International University Press, 1961.

Boston Women's Health Collective. *Our Bodies, Ourselves.* New York: Simon and Schuster, 1976.

Bowlby, John. *Attachment and Loss.* New York: Basic Books, 1969.

———. "Process of Mourning." *Int. J. Psychoanal.* 42 (1961):317–340.

Brown, Norman O. *Life against Death.* New York: Vintage Books, 1959.

Cain, A. C., M. E. Erikson, I. Fast, and R. A. Vaughn. "Children's Disturbed Reactions to Their Mother's Miscarriage." *Psychosomatic Medicine* 24 (1964): 58–66.

Chodorow, Nancy. *The Reproduction of Mothering.* Berkeley: University of California Press, 1978.

Corney, R. T., and F. T. Horton, Jr. "Pathological Grief Following Spontaneous Abortion." *Am. J. of Psychiatry* 131 (1974):825–827.

Costello, A., et al. "Perinatal Grief and Loss." *J. Perinatol.* 8 (1988):361–370.

Deutsch, Helene. *Motherhood. The Psychology of Women,* vol. 2. New York: Grune and Stratton, 1945.

Engel, George L. "Grief and Grieving." *Am. J. Nursing,* 64 (1964):93–98.

Feinbloom, Richard I. *Pregnancy, Birth, and the Newborn Baby.* New York: Dell, 1972.

Friedman, Rochelle R., and Karen A. Cohen. "Emotional Reactions to the Miscarriage of a Consciously Desired Pregnancy." In *The Woman Patient,* ed. Malkah Notman and Carol Nadelson, vol. 3. New York: Plenum Press, 1982.

———. "The Peer Support Group: A Model for Dealing with the Emotional Aspects of Miscarriage." *Group* 4 (1980):42–48.

Furlong, R. M. "Grief in the Perinatal Period." *Obstet. Gynecol.* 61 (1983):497.

Gardner, S., and G. Merenstein. "Helping Families Deal With Perinatal Loss." *Neonatal Network* (1986).

Gaylin, Willard. *Caring.* New York: Avon, 1976.

Gradstein, Bonnie D., and Rhoda Levitt. *Guidelines for Pregnancy Counseling.* San Francisco: San Francisco Interagency Pregnancy Council, 1975. Distributed by Department of Health, Office of Planning.

Graham, M. A., et al. "Factors Affecting Psychological Adjustment to a Fetal Death." *Am. J. Obs. and Gyn.* 157 (1987):254–257.

Grimm, E. R. "Psychological Investigation of Habitual Abortion." *Psychosomatic Medicine* 24 (1962):369.

———. "Psychological Tension in Pregnancy." *Psychosomatic Medicine* 23 (1961):520–527.

Grossman, Frances Kaplan, Lois S. Eichler, Susan A. Winickoff, et al. *Pregnancy, Birth, and Parenthood.* San Francisco: Jossey-Bass, 1980.

Hamburg, D. A., and J. E. Adams. "A Perspective on Coping Behavior: Seeking and Utilizing Information in Major Transitions." *Arch. Gen. Psychiat.* 17 (1967):277–284.

Ilse, S., and L. Burns. *Empty Arms: Coping After Miscarriage, Stillbirth and Infant Death.* P.O. Box 165, Long Lake, Minn. 55356, 1982.

Jessner, L., E. Weigert, and J. L. Foy. "The Development of Parental Attitudes during Pregnancy." In *Parenthood: Its Psychology and Psychopathology*, ed. James Anthony and Therese Benedek. Boston: Little, Brown, 1970.

Jessner, Lucie. "On Becoming a Mother." In *Conditio Humana*, ed. Walter von Baeyer and Richard M. Griffith. New York: Springer-Verlag, 1966.

Josselyn, Irene M. "Cultural Forces, Motherliness and Fatherliness." *Am. J. Orthopsychiatry* 26 (1945):264–271.

Kaij, L., A. Malmquist, and A. Nilsson. "Psychiatric Aspects of Spontaneous Abortion. II. The Importance of Bereavement, Attachment and Neurosis in Early Life." *J. of Psychosomatic Res.* 13 (1969):53–59.

Kennell, John H., Howard Slyter, and Marshall H. Klaus. "Mourning Response of Parents to the Death of a Newborn Infant." *NEJM* 283 (1970):344–349.

Kestenberg, Judith S. "Regression and Reintegration in Pregnancy." *J. Am. Psychoanal. Assn.* 24 (1976): supplement, *Female Psychology.*

Kirk, E. P. "Psychological Effects and Management of Perinatal Loss." *Am. J. Obs. and Gyn.* 149 (1984):46–51.

Klaus, Marshall H., and John H. Kennell. *Maternal-Infant Bonding.* St. Louis: Mosby, 1976.

Lennane, K. Jean and R. John. "Alleged Psychogenic Disorders in Women: A Possible Manifestation of Sexual Prejudice." *NEJM* 288 (1973).

Leon, I. G. "Psychodynamics of Perinatal Loss." *Psychiatry* 9 (1986):312–324.

Lindemann, Erich. "Symptomatology and Management of Acute Grief." *Am J. of Psychiatry* 101 (1944):141.

McBride, A. B. *The Growth and Development of Mothers.* New York: Harper and Row, 1974.

McDonald, Ronald L. "The Role of Emotional Factors in Obstetric Complications: A Review." *Psychosomatic Medicine* 30 (1968):222–237.

Malmquist, A., L. Kaij, and A. Nilsson. "Psychiatric Aspects of Spontaneous Abortion. I. A Matched Control Study of Women with Living Children." *J. of Psychosomatic Res.* 13 (1969):45–51.

Menning, Barbara Eck. *Infertility: A Guide for the Childless Couple.* Englewood Cliffs: Prentice-Hall, 1977.

Michel-Wolfromm, H. "The Psychological Factor in Spontaneous Abortion." *J. of Psychosomatic Res.* 12 (1968):67–71.

Miller, Rita S. "The Social Construction and Reconstruction of Physiologic Events: Acquiring the Pregnancy Identity." In Norman K. Denzin (ed.), *Studies in Symbolic Interaction*, vol. 1. (1978), pp. 181–204.

Parkes, C. Murray. "The Nature of Grief." *Int. J. of Psychiatry* 3 (1967):435–438.

Pohlman, Edward. *The Psychology of Birth Planning.* Cambridge, Mass.: Schenkman, 1969.

Pollock, G. "Mourning and Adaptation." *Int. J. Psychoanal.* 42 (1961):341–361.

Russell, Keith P. *Eastman's Expectant Motherhood.* 7th ed. Boston: Little, Brown, 1980.

Sander, W. "Adaptive Relationships in Early Mother-Child Interaction." *J. Am Acad. Child Psychiatry,* 3 (1964):231–265.

Seibel, Machelle, and William L. Graves. "The Psychological Implications of Spontaneous Abortion." *J. of Reproductive Medicine* 25 (1980):161–165.

Sherman, Julia A. "Pregnancy." In *On the Psychology of Woman: A Survey of Empirical Studies.* Illinois: Charles C. Thomas, 1973.

Siggins, Lorraine D. "Mourning: A Critical Survey of the Literature." *Int. J. Psychoanal.* 47 (1966):14–25.

Simon, N. M., P. Rothman, J. T. Goff, et al. "Psychological Factors Related to Spontaneous and Therapeutic Abortion." *Am. J. Obs. and Gyn.* 104 (1969):799–806.

Solnit, Albert J., and Mary H. Stark. *Mourning and the Birth of a Defective Child. Psychoanalytic Study of the Child,* vol. 16. New York: International University Press (1961).

Stack, Jack M. "Spontaneous Abortion and Grieving." *American Family Physician* 21 (1980):99–102.

Toedter, L. J., et al. "The Perinatal Grief Scale: Development and Initial Validation." *Am. J. Orthopsychiatry* 58 (1988):435–449.

Tupper, C., et al. "The Problem of Spontaneous Abortion." *Am. J. Obs. and Gyn.* 73 (1957):313.

Wathen, N. C. "Perinatal Bereavement." *Brit. J. Obs. and Gyn.* 149 (1984):46–51.

Winnicott, D. W. "The Theory of Parent-Infant Relationship." In *The Maturational Process and the Facilitating Environment,* ed. D. W. Winnicott. New York: International University Press, 1965.

Yalom, Irvin D., et al. "Postpartum Blues Syndrome." *Arch. Gen. Psychiatry* 18 (1968): 16–27.

Zeanah, C. "Adaptation Following Perinatal Loss: A Critical Review." *J. Am. Acad. Child and Adolesc. Psychiatry* 28 (1989):467–480.

MISCARRIAGE

Alberman, E., et al. "Previous Reproductive History in Mothers Presenting with Spontaneous Abortions." *Brit. J. Obs. and Gyn.* 82 (1975):366.

Assali, Nicholas S., ed. *Pathophysiology of Gestation,* vol. 2. New York: Academic Press, 1972.

Barnes, Ann B., et al. "Fertility and Outcome of Pregnancy in Women Exposed in Utero to Diethylstilbestrol." *NEJM* 302, No. 11 (1980):609–613.

Bennett, M. J., and R. H. J. Kerr-Wilson. "Evaluation of Threatened Abortion by Ultrasound." *Int. J. Gyn. and Obs.* 17 (1980):382–384.

Byrd, J. Rogers, et al. "Cytogenic Findings in Fifty-five Couples with Recurrent Fetal Wastage." *Fertility and Sterility* 28 (1977):246–250.

Cain, Albert C., et al. "Children's Disturbed Reactions to Their Mother's Miscarriage." *Psychosomatic Medicine* 26 (1964):58–66.

Carr, D. H. "Chromosome Anomalies as a Cause of Spontaneous Abortion." *Am. J. Obs. and Gyn.* 97 (1967):283–293.

———. "Genetic Basis of Abortion." *Annual Rev. of Genetics* 5 (1971):64.

Clapp, Diane. "Luteal Phase Defect." *RESOLVE Newsletter,* September 1980.

———. "T-Mycoplasm: Its Role in Infertility and Miscarriage." *RESOLVE Newsletter,* June 1979.

Danforth, David N., ed. *Obstetrics and Gynecology,* 3rd ed. New York: Harper and Row, 1977.

Fabricant, Jill D., et al. "Cytogenetic Abnormalities in Spontaneous Abortion." In *Management of High Risk Pregnancy,* ed. John T. Queenan. Oradell: Medical Economics, 1980.

———. "Genetic Studies on Spontaneous Abortion." *Contemporary Obs. and Gyn.* 11 (1978):73–78.

Friedman, T., and D. Gath. "The Psychiatric Consequences of Spontaneous Abortion." *Brit. J. Psychiatry* 155 (1989): 810–813.

Glass, Robert H., ed. *Office Gynecology,* 2nd ed. Baltimore: Williams and Wilkins, 1981.

Glass, Robert H., and Mitchell S. Golbus. "Habitual Abortion." *Fertility and Sterility* 29 (1978):257–265.

Gnarpe, H., and J. Friberg. "Mycoplasma and Human Reproduction Failure." *Am. J. Obs. and Gyn.* 114 (1972):727.

Goldstein, Donald P., and Merle J. Berger. "Reproductive Failure in DES-Exposed Women." *RESOLVE Newsletter,* June 1980.

Grimm, Elaine R. "Psychological Investigation of Habitual Abortion." *Psychosomatic Medicine* 24 (1962):369–378.

Grimm, Elaine R., and Wanda R. Venet. "The Relationship of Emotional Adjustment and Attitudes to the Course and Outcome of Pregnancy." *Psychosomatic Medicine* 28 (1966):34–49.

Guerrero, R., and O. I. Rojas. "Spontaneous Abortion and Aging of Human Ova and Spermatozoa." *NEJM* 293 (1975):573.

Hall, R. C., et al. "Grief Following Spontaneous Abortion." *Psychiat. Clin. North Am.* 10 (1987):405–420.

Hamilton, S. M. "Should Follow-up Be Provided After Miscarriage?" *Brit. J. Obs. and Gyn.* 96 (1989):743–745.

Hayton, A. "Miscarriage and Delayed Depression." *The Lancet* (April 9, 1988):834.

Hertiz, A. T., and R. G. Livingstone. "Spontaneous Threatened and Habitual Abortion: Their Prognosis and Treatment." *NEJM* 230 (1944):798.

Ilse, S., and L. Burns. *Miscarriage — A Shattered Dream.* P.O. Box 165, Long Lake, Minn. 55356, 1985.

James, William H. "The Problem of Spontaneous Abortion." *Am. J. Obs. and Gyn.* 85 (1963):38–40.

Kajii, Tadashi, and Ariane Ferrier. "Cytogenetics of Aborters and Abortuses." *Am. J. Obs. and Gyn.* 131 (1978):33.

Kline, J. "Smoking a Risk Factor for Spontaneous Abortion." *NEJM* 297 (1977):793–796.

Malmquist, A., L. Kaij, and A. Nilsson. "Psychiatric Aspects of Spontaneous Abortion. I. A Matched Control Study of Women with Living Children." *J. of Psychosomatic Res.* 13 (1969):45–51.

Menning, Barbara Eck, and Diane Clapp. "The Emotional Impact of Miscarriage." *RESOLVE Newsletter,* September 1979.

Michel-Wolfromm, H. "The Psychological Factor in Habitual Abortion." *J. of Psychosomatic Res.* 12 (1968):67–71.

Newton, Niels. "Emotions of Pregnancy." *Clinical Obs. and Gyn.* 6 (1963):638–668.

Niswander, Kenneth R. *Obstetrics: Essentials of Clinical Practice,* 2nd ed. Boston: Little, Brown, 1981.

Patterson, Sam P., and William T. Black, Jr. "When Women Habitually Abort." *Postgraduate Medicine* 43 (1968):59–66.

Schweditsch, M. O. "Hormonal Considerations in Early Normal Pregnancy and Blighted Ovum Syndrome." *Fertility and Sterility* 31 (1979):252–257.

Seibel, Machelle, and William L. Graves. "The Psychological Implications of Spontaneous Abortion." *J. of Reproductive Medicine* 25 (1980):161–165.

Sher, G. "Induction of Labor Following Intrauterine Death with Intra-amniotic Hyperosmolar Urea and Prostaglandin F2 α: Evaluation of Placental Endocrine Function and Changes in Coagulation Parameters." *Am. J. Obs and Gyn.* 134 (1979):493–497.

Simon, N. M., et al. "Psychological Factors Related to Spontaneous and Therapeutic Abortion." *Am. J. Obs and Gyn.* 104 (1969):799–806.

Speroff, L., R. H. Glass, and N. Kase. *Clinical Gynecologic Endocrinology and Infertility,* 2nd ed. Baltimore: Williams and Wilkins, 1978.

Stack, Jack. "Spontaneous Abortion and Grieving." *Am. Family Physician* 21 (1980):99–102.

Surgeon General's Advisory on Alcohol and Pregnancy. *FDA Drug Bulletin* 11 (July 1981).

Taylor, E. Stewart, ed. *Beck's Obstetrical Practice and Fetal Medicine.* Baltimore: Williams and Wilkins, 1976.

Tho, Phung T., J. R. Byrd, and P. G. McDonough. "Etiologies and Subsequent Reproductive Performance of 100 Couples with Recurrent Abortion." *Fertility and Sterility* 32 (1979):389–395.

Tupper, C., et al. "The Problem of Spontaneous Abortion." *Am. J. Obs and Gyn.* 73 (1957):313–321.

Wall-Haas, C. "Women's Perceptions of First Trimester Spontaneous Abortion." *JOGNN* (January–February 1985):51–52.

Weathersbee, P. S., et al. "Caffeine in Pregnancy." *Postgraduate Medicine* 62 (1977):64–69.

STILLBIRTH

"The Abhorrence of Stillbirth." *The Lancet* (1977):1188–1190.

Beard, R. W., et al. "Help for Parents after Stillbirth." *Brit. Medical J.* 1 (1978):172–173.

Beischer, N. A., and E. V. Mackay. "Ultrasonic Echography." In *Obstetrics and the Newborn.* Philadelphia: Saunders, 1976.

Bourne, Stanford. "The Psychological Effects of Stillbirths on the Doctor." *Proceedings,* Third International Congress of Psychosomatic Medicine in Obstetrics and Gynaecology, London, 1971, pp. 333–334.

———. "The Psychological Effects of Stillbirths on Women and Their Doctors." *J. Royal College of General Practitioners* 16 (1968):103–112.

Brans, Y. W., et al. "Perinatal Mortality in a Large Perinatal Center: Five-Year Review of 31,000 Births." *Am. J. Obs. and Gyn.* 148 (1984):284–289.

Breuer, Judith. "Sharing a Tragedy." *Am. J. Nursing* 76 (1976):758–759.

Clarke, Michael. "Depression in Women after Perinatal Death." *The Lancet* 1 (1979):916–917.

Condon, John. "Management of Established Pathological Grief Reaction After Stillbirth." *Am. J. of Psychiatry* 143 (1986):987–992.

Cullberg, J. "Mental Reactions of Women to Perinatal Death." *Proceedings*, Third International Congress of Psychosomatic Medicine in Obstetrics and Gynaecology, London, 1971, pp. 326–329.

Danforth, David N., ed. *Obstetrics and Gynecology*, 3rd ed. New York: Harper and Row, 1977.

Dunlop, Joyce. "Bereavement Reaction Following Stillbirth." *The Practitioner* 222 (1979):115–118.

"Easing the Pain and Grief of Stillbirth." *Nursing Mirror* 146 (June 1, 1978): 38–41.

Engel, George L. "Grief and Grieving." *Am. J. Nursing* 64 (1964):93–98.

Fedrick, Jean, and Philippa Adelstein. "Influences of Pregnancy Spacing on Outcome of Pregnancy." *Brit. J. Medicine* 29 (1973):753–756.

Giles, P. F. H. "Reactions of Women to Perinatal Death." *Australian and New Zealand J. of Obs. and Gyn.* 10 (1970):207–210.

Goplerud, Clifford P. "Bleeding in Late Pregnancy." In *Obstetrics and Gynecology*, 3rd ed., ed. David N. Danforth. New York: Harper and Row, 1977, pp. 378–387.

Hallett, Elizabeth R. "Birth and Grief." *Birth and the Family J.* 1 (1974):18–22.

Hardgrove, Carol, and Louise Warrick. "How Shall We Tell the Children?" *Am. J. Nursing* 74 (1974):448–450.

Jolly, Hugh. "Family Reactions to Child Bereavement." *Proceedings* of the Royal Society of Medicine 69 (1976):835–842.

———. "Loss of a Baby." *Australian Pediatric J.* 14 (1978):3–5.

Kennell, John H., et al. "The Mourning Response of Parents to the Death of a Newborn Infant." *NEJM* 283 (1976):344–346.

Knapp, Ronald J., and Larry G. Peppers. "Doctor-Patient Relationships in Fetal/Infant Death Encounters." *J. Medical Education* 54 (1979):775–780.

Kotzwinkle, William. "Swimmer in the Secret Sea." *Redbook Magazine*, July 1974.

Laursen, N. H., et al. "Management of Intrauterine Fetal Death with Prostaglandins E_2 Vaginal Suppositories." *Am. J. Obs. and Gyn.* 137 (1980):753–757.

Lewis, B. Victor, et al. "Vaginal Breech Delivery or Cesarean Section?" *Am. J. Obs. and Gyn.* 134 (1979):615–618.

Lewis, Emanuel. "The Management of Stillbirth: Coping with an Unreality." *The Lancet* 2 (1976):619–620.

———. "Mourning by the Family after a Stillbirth or Neonatal Death." *Archives of Disease in Childhood* 54 (1979):303–306.

———. "Reactions to Stillbirth." *Proceedings*, Third International Congress of Psychosomatic Medicine in Obstetrics and Gynaecology, London, 1971, pp. 323–325.

Lewis, Emanuel, and Anne Page. "Failure to Mourn a Stillborn: An Overlooked Catastrophe." *Brit. J. Medical Psychology* 51 (1978):237–241.

Lindemann, Erich. "Symptomatology and Management of Acute Grief." *Am. J. of Psychiatry* 101 (1944):141–148.

Mann, Leon L. "Modern Management of the Breech Delivery." *Am. J. Obs. and Gyn.* 134 (1979):611–614.

Moore, T. R., and K. Piacquado. "A Prospective Evaluation of Fetal Movement Screening to Reduce the Incidence of Antepartum Feat Death." *Am. J. Obs. and Gyn.* 160 (1989):1075–1080.

Newton, Michael. "Other Complications of Labor." In *Obstetrics and Gynecology*, 3rd ed., ed. David L. Danforth. New York: Harper and Row, 1977.

Parkes, C. Murray. "The Nature of Grief." *Int. J. of Psychiatry* 3 (1967):435–438.

Poznanski, Elva Orlow. "The Replacement Child: A Saga of Unresolved Parental Grief." *J. Pediatrics* 81 (1972):1191–1193.

Ross, Tamara. "Stillbirth: A New Approach." Interview with Hugh Jolly, *Nursing Mirror* 143 (1976):40–41.

Rowe, J., et al. "Followup: Families Who Experience a Perinatal Death." *J. Pediatrics* 62 (1978):166–170.

Seitz, Pauline M., and Louise H. Warrick. "Perinatal Death: The Grieving Mother." *Am. J. Nursing* 74 (1974):2028–2033.

Sher, G. "Induction of Labor Following Intrauterine Death with Intra-amniotic Hypersmolar Urea and Prostaglandin F_2 α: Evaluation of Placental Endocrine Function and Changes in Coagulation Parameters." *Am. J. Obs. and Gyn.* 134 (1979).

Sonstegard, Lois, et al. "The Grieving Nurse." *Am. J. Nursing* 76 (1976):1490–1492.

Speck, William T. "Commentary: The Tragedy of Stillbirth." *J. Pediatrics* 93 (1978):869–870.

Taylor, E. Stewart, ed. *Beck's Obstetrical Practice and Fetal Medicine.* Baltimore: Williams and Wilkins, 1976.

Wolff, John R. "The Emotional Reaction to a Stillbirth." *Proceedings,* Third International Congress of Psychosomatic Medicine in Obstetrics and Gynaecology, London, 1971, pp. 330–332.

Wolff, John R., et al. "The Emotional Reaction to a Stillbirth." *Am J. Obs. and Gyn.* 108 (1970):73–77.

Worlow, Dorothy. "What Do You Say When the Baby Is Stillborn?" *RN* 41 (1978):74.

ECTOPIC PREGNANCY

Bender, S. "Fertility after Tubal Pregnancy." *Brit. J. Obs. and Gyn.* 63 (1956):400.

Boyd, J. E., and E. M. Holt. "Tubal Sterility, Patency Tests, and Results of Operation." *Brit. J. Obs. and Gyn.* 80 (1973):142.

Bukovsky, I., et al. "Conservative Surgery for Tubal Pregnancy." *Obs. and Gyn.* 53 (1979):709–711.

DeVore, N., and K. Baldwin. "Ectopic Pregnancy on the Rise." *Am. J. Nursing* 86 (1986):674–678.

Franklin, E. W., III, A. M. Zeiderman, and P. Laemmle. "Tubal Ectopic Pregnancy: Etiology and Obstetric and Gynecologic Sequelae." *Am. J. Obs. and Gyn.* 117 (1973):220.

Glass, Robert H. *Office Gynecology*, 2nd ed. Baltimore: Williams and Wilkins, 1981.

Hallatt, J. G. "Repeat Ectopic Pregnancy: A Study of 123 Consecutive Cases." *Am. J. Obs. and Gyn.* 122 (1975):520.

Kitchin, James D., III, et al. "Ectopic Pregnancy: Current Clinical Trends." *Am. J. Obs. and Gyn.* 134 (1979):870.

Osguthorpe, N. "Ectopic Pregnancy." *JOGNN* 16 (1987):36–41.

Schenker, J. G., et al. "Fertility after Tubal Pregnancy." *Surg. Gyn. and Obs.* 135 (1972):74–76.

Schoen, J. A., and R. J. Nowak. "Repeat Ectopic Pregnancy." *Obs. and Gyn.* 45 (1975):542–546.

Skulj, V., Z. Pavlic, C. Stoilkovic, et al. "Conservative Operative Treatment of Tubal Pregnancy." *Fertility and Sterility* 15 (1964):634.

Toaff, R. "Disturbances of Gestational Potency." In Charles A. Joel, *Fertility Disturbances in Men and Women.* New York: S. Karger, 1971.

PRENATAL DIAGNOSIS

"Afterwords." Prenatal Diagnostic Center, 80 Hayden Ave., Lexington, Mass. 02173.

Black, R. B. "Prenatal Diagnosis and Fetal Loss: Psychosocial Consequences and Professional Responsibilities." *Am. J. of Medical Genetics* 35 (1990):586–587.

Blatt, R. *Prenatal Tests: What They Are, Their Benefits and Risks, and How to Decide Whether to Have Them or Not.* New York: Vintage Books, 1988.

Blumberg, B., et al. "The Psychological Sequelae of Abortion Performed for a Genetic Indication." *Am. J. Obs. and Gyn.* 122 (1975).

Donnai, P., et al. "Attitudes of Patients After Genetic Termination of Pregnancy." *Brit. Medical J.* 282 (1981): 621.

Drotar, D., et al. "The Adaptation of Parents to the Birth of an Infant with a Congenital Malformation." *Pediatrics* 56 (1975):711–716.

Faden, R. R., et al. "Prenatal Screening and Pregnant Women's Attitudes Towards the Abortion of Defective Fetuses." *Am. J. Pub. Health* 77 (1987): 288–290.

Firth, H. V., et al. "Severe Limb Abnormalities After Chorion Villus Sampling at 55–60 Days' Gestation," *The Lancet* (March 30, 1991): 762–763.

Hodge, S. E. "Waiting for the Amniocentesis." *NEJM* 320 (1989):63–64.

Jones, O. W., et al. "Parental Response to Midtrimester Therapeutic Abortion Following Amniocentesis." *Prenatal Diagnosis* 4 (1984):249–256.

Meryash, D. L. "Perception of Burden Among At-Risk Women of Raising a Child with Fragile-X Syndrome." *Clin. Genet.* 36 (1989):15–24.

Oustifine, J. M. "Abortion After Amniocentesis." Master's thesis, MGH Institute of Health Professions, 1990.

Pauker, S. G., et al. "The Effect of Private Attitudes on Public Policy: Prenatal Screening for Neural Tube Defects As a Prototype." *Med. Decis. Making* 1 (1981):103–114.

"Prenatal Genetic Diagnosis." Prenatal Diagnostic Center, 80 Hayden Ave., Lexington, Mass. 02173.

Richards, M. P. M. "Social and Ethical Problems of Fetal Diagnosis and Screening." *Reproductive and Infant Psychology* 7 (1989).

Rothman, B. K. *The Tentative Pregnancy: Prenatal Diagnosis and the Future of Motherhood.* New York: Viking, 1986.

Smith, J. D. "Down's Syndrome, Amniocentesis, and Abortion: Prevention or Elimination?" *Ment. Retard.* 19 (1981):8–11.

MULTIPLE LOSSES

Berger, M., and D. Goldstein. "Impaired Reproductive Performance in DES-Exposed Women." *Obs. and Gyn.* 55 (1980):25–27.

Danforth, David N., ed. *Obstetrics and Gynecology*, 3rd ed. New York: Harper and Row, 1977.

Glass, R. H., and M. S. Golbus. "Habitual Abortion." *Fertility and Sterility* 29 (1978):257–265.

Grimm, Elaine R. "Psychological Investigation of Habitual Abortion." *Psychosomatic Medicine* 24 (1962):369–378.

Hendin, David, and Joan Marks. *The Genetic Connection.* New York: Signet, 1979.

Hertz, Dan G. "Rejection of Motherhood." *Psychosomatics* 14 (1973):241–244.

Mazor, M. "The Problem of Infertility." In *The Woman Patient*, vol. 1, ed. Malkah Notman and Carol Nadelson. New York: Plenum Press, 1978.

———. "Barren Couples." *Psychology Today*, May 1979.

Menning, Barbara Eck. *Infertility: A Guide for the Childless Couple.* Englewood Cliffs, N.J.: Prentice-Hall, 1978.

———. "Counseling Infertile Couples." *Contemporary Obs. and Gyn.* 13 (1979):101–108.

———. "The Emotional Needs of Infertile Couples." *Fertility and Sterility* 34 (1980):313–319.

Niswander, Kenneth R. *Obstetrics: Essentials of Clinical Practice*, 2nd ed. Boston: Little, Brown, 1981.

Patterson, Sam P., and William T. Black, Jr. "When Women Habitually Abort." *Postgraduate Medicine* 43 (1968):59–66.

Rosenfeld, D. L., and E. Mitchell. "Treating the Emotional Aspects of Infertility: Counseling Services in an Infertility Clinic." *Am. J. Obs. and Gyn.* 135 (1979):177–180.

Speroff, L., R. H. Glass, and N. G. Kase. *Clinical Gynecologic Endocrinology and Infertility*, 2nd ed. Baltimore: Williams and Wilkins, 1978.

Stangel, John J. *Fertility and Conception: An Essential Guide for Childless Couples.* New York: Paddington Press, 1979.

Taylor, E. Stewart, ed. *Beck's Obstetrical Practice and Fetal Medicine.* Baltimore: Williams and Wilkins, 1976.

Tho, Phung T., J. Rogers Byrd, and Paul G. McDonough. "Etiologies and Subsequent Reproductive Performance of 100 Couples with Recurrent Abortion." *Fertility and Sterility* 32 (1979):389–395.

THE NEW ASSISTED REPRODUCTIVE TECHNOLOGIES

Corson, S. L., et al. "Outcome in 242 *In Vitro* Fertilization Embryo Replacement or Gamete Intrafallopian Transfer-Induced Pregnancies." *Fertility and Sterility* 514 (1989):644–650.

Glass, R. H., and R. J. Ericsson. *Getting Pregnant in the 1980s: New Advances in Infertility, Treatment and Sex Preselection.* Berkeley: University of California Press, 1982.

Lasker, J., and S. Borg. *In Search of Parenthood.* Boston: Beacon Press, 1987.

Liebmann-Smith, J. *In Pursuit of Pregnancy.* New York: Newmarket Press, 1987.

Mazor, M., and H. F. Simons. eds., *Infertility — Medical, Emotional and Social Considerations.* New York: Human Sciences Press, 1984.

Newton, C. R., et al. "Psychological Assessment and Follow-up After *In Vitro* Fertilization: Assessing the Impact of Failure." *Fertility and Sterility* 54 (1990):879–886.

Romeu, A., et al. "Results of *In Vitro* Fertilization Attempts in Women 40 Years of Age and Older: The Norfolk Experience." *Fertility and Sterility* 47 (1987):130–136.

Soules, M. R. "The *In Vitro* Fertilization Pregnancy Rate: Let's Be Honest with One Another." *Fertility and Sterility* 43 (1985):511–513.

Tilton, N., et al. *Making Miracles: In Vitro Fertilization.* Garden City, N.Y.: Doubleday, 1985.

Williams, L. "It's Going to Work for Me: Responses to Failures of IVF." *Birth* 15 (1988):153–156.

Yovick, J. and E. W. "The Relative Chance of Pregnancy Following Tubal or Uterine Transfer Procedure." *Fertility and Sterility* 49 (1988):859–864.

Yulsman, T. "A Little Help for Creation." *New York Times Magazine,* October 7, 1990, 22–29.

THE HUSBAND'S EXPERIENCE

Freeman, T. "Pregnancy as a Precipitant of Mental Illness in Men." *Brit. J. Medical Psychol.* 24 (1951):49.

"Grieving after Spontaneous Abortion Often Unrecognized." *Obs. Gyn. News* 14 (1981):31.

Group for the Advancement of Psychiatry, Committee in Public Education. *The Joys and Sorrows of Parenthood.* New York: Charles Scribner's Sons, 1973.

Jarvis, W. "Some Effects of Pregnancy and Childbirth on Men." *J. Am Psychoanal. Assn.* 10 (1962):689–700.

Josselyn, Irene M. "Cultural Forces, Motherliness and Fatherliness." *Am. J. Orthopsychiatry* 26 (1956):264–271.

Kennell, John H., Howard Slyter, and Marshall H. Klaus. "The Mourning Response of Parents to the Death of a Newborn." *NEJM* 283 (1970): 344–349.

Pleck, Joseph H., and Jack Sawyer, eds. *Men and Masculinity.* Englewood Cliffs, N.J.: Prentice-Hall, 1974.

Zilboorg, Gregory. "Depressive Reactions Related to Parenthood." *Am. J. of Psychiatry* 10 (1931):927–962.

FAMILY AND FRIENDS: REACTIONS OF AND REACTIONS TO

Cain, Albert C., et al. "Children's Disturbed Reactions to Their Mothers' Miscarriage." *Psychosomatic Medicine* 24 (1964):58–66.

Cain, Albert C., I. Fast, and M. E. Erickson. "Children's Disturbed Reactions to the Death of a Sibling." *Am J. Orthopsychiatry* 34 (1964):741–752.

Cain, A. C., et al. "On Replacing a Child." *J. Am Acad. Child Psychiatry* 3 (1964):443–456.

Hardgrove, Carol, and Louise H. Warrick. "How Shall We Tell the Children?" *Am. J. Nursing* 74 (1974):448–450.

Jolly, Hugh. "Family Reactions to Child Bereavement." *Proceedings*, Royal Society of Medicine 69 (1976):835–842.

———. "Loss of a Baby." *Australian Pediatric J.* 14 (1978):3–5.

Klaus, Marshall H., and John H. Kennell. *Maternal-Infant Bonding*. St. Louis: Mosby, 1976.

Lewis, Emanuel. "Mourning by the Family after a Stillbirth or Neonatal Death." *Archives of Disease of Childhood* 54 (1979):303–306.

———. "Reactions to Stillbirth." *Proceedings*, International Congress of Psychosomatic Medicine in Obstetrics and Gynaecology, Third International Congress. Basel: Karger, 1972.

Nagera, Humberto. "Children's Reactions to the Death of Important Objects: A Development Approach." In *The Psychoanalytical Study of the Child*, vol. 25. New York: International University Press, 1970.

BOOKS ON DEATH FOR CHILDREN (AND PARENTS)

Primary Grades and Preschool
De Bruyn, M. G. *The Beaver Who Wouldn't Die*. Chicago: Follett, 1975.
Fassler, Joan. *My Grandpa Died Today*. New York: Behavioral Publications, 1971.
Viorst, Judith. *The Tenth Good Thing about Barney*. New York: Atheneum, 1971.

Children 10 to 14 Years Old
Miles, Betty. *The Trouble with Thirteen*. New York: Knopf, 1979.
Paterson, Katherine. *The Bridge to Terabithia*. New York: Crowell, 1977.

Parents and Children
Zim, Herbert S., and Sonia Bleeker. *Life and Death*. New York: Morrow, 1970.

Parents
Grollman, Earl. *Explaining Death to Children*. Boston: Beacon Press, 1969.
Rudolph, Marguerita. *Should the Children Know? Encounters with Death in the Lives of Children*. New York: Schocken, 1978.
Wolf, Anna W. M., ed. *Helping Your Child to Understand Death*. Child Study Association of America, 1958.

PLANNING FOR THE FUTURE

"AMA Labels Marijuana as Dangerous Drug." *Psychiatric News*, April 17, 1981.
Bernard, J. *The Future of Motherhood*. New York: Penguin, 1975.
Caplan, L. *An Open Adoption*. Boston: Houghton Mifflin, 1991.
Clarren, Sterling K., and David W. Smith. "The Fetal Alcohol Syndrome." *NEJM* 298 (1978):1063–1067.

Daniels, P., and K. Weingarten. "A New Look at the Medical Risks in Late Childbearing." *Women and Health* 4 (1979):5–35.

Davis, D., et al. "Postponing Pregnancy After Perinatal Death: Perspectives on Doctor Advice." *J. Am. Acad. Child and Adolesc. Psychiatry* 28 (1989):481–487.

Fedrick, Jean, and Philippa Adelstein. "Influence of Pregnancy Spacing on Outcome of Pregnancy." *British Medical J.* 4 (1973):753–756.

Harrison, Mary. *Infertility: A Guide for Couples.* Boston: Houghton Mifflin, 1979.

Menning, Barbara Eck. *Infertility: A Guide for Childless Couples.* Englewood Cliffs, N.J.: Prentice-Hall, 1978.

Perkins, Richard P. "Sexual Behavior and Response in Relation to Complications of Pregnancy." *Am. J. Obs. and Gyn.* 134 (1979):498–505.

Phipps, S. "The Subsequent Pregnancy After Stillbirth: Anticipatory Parenthood in the Face of Uncertainty." *Int. J. of Psychiatry in Medicine* 15 (1985–86):243–264.

Poznanski, Elva Orlow. "The Replacement Child: A Saga of Unresolved Parental Grief." *J. Pediatrics* 81 (1972):1190–1193.

"Pregnancy: The Ultimate Goal." *RESOLVE Newsletter,* Sept. 1980.

Speroff, L., R. H. Glass, and N. G. Kase. *Clinical Gynecologic Endocrinology and Infertility,* 2nd ed. Baltimore: Williams and Wilkins, 1978.

Surgeon General's Advisory on Alcohol and Pregnancy. *FDA Drug Bulletin,* 11 (1981):1.

ADOPTION

Arms, Suzanne. *Adoption: A Handful of Hope.* Berkeley: Celestial Arts, 1990.

———. *To Love and Let Go.* New York: Alfred A. Knopf, 1983.

Dywasuk, Colette T. *Adoption: Is It For You?* New York: Harper and Row, 1973.

Gilman, Lois. *The Adoption Resource Book.* New York: Harper and Row, 1984, 1987.

Gradstein, B., M. Gradstein, and R. Glass. "Private Adoption." *Fertility and Sterility* 37 (1982).

Lifton, Betty Jean. *Lost and Found.* New York: Dial Press, 1979, 1983.

McNamara, Joan. *The Adoption Advisor.* New York: Hawthorne Books, 1975.

Martin, Cynthia. *Beating the Adoption Game.* New York: Harcourt Brace Jovanovich, 1988.

Melina, Lois Ruskai. *Making Sense of Adoption.* New York: Harper and Row, 1989.

Paul, Ellen. *Adoption Choices.* Detroit: Visible Ink Press, 1991.

Raymond, Louise. *Adoption and After.* New York: Harper and Row, 1974.

Rillera, Mary Jo, and Sharon, Kaplan. *Cooperative Adoption: A Handbook.* Westminster: Triadoption Publications, 1984, 1985.

Silber, Kathleen, and Patricia Martinez Dorner. *Children of Open Adoption.* San Antonio: Corona Publishing, 1990.

Sorosky, Arthur D., A. Baran, and R. Pannor. *The Adoption Triangle.* New York: Anchor, 1978.

Index